Introduction

I can't tell you how thrilled I am that you are reading this book right now. It means that you are either thinking about trying for a baby and want to get your body in the best shape possible, or that you are already pregnant (if so, I send my huge congratulations).

Blooming Delicious came about through necessity and completely organically. When my husband and I started to think about the future and the idea of trying for a baby, I knew that it was really important to prepare my body in the best way possible, both nutritionally and physically, to give a new baby the best fighting chance to grow healthy and strong during those long nine months inside me.

I didn't want a new diet or regime to take over my life, adding extra pressure and stress to the process of 'trying' for a baby. I wanted to take the most natural route possible and let nature take its course, while ensuring I was doing all the right things in nutritional terms.

I did what most of us do in this day and age when we want something: jumped on to Amazon. I was looking for a pregnancy cookbook that was easy to follow and accessible to a busy working professional foodie like me. I found lots of nutritionally focused cookery books,

but, although they were very interesting to read, they didn't exactly inspire the chef in me.

So I made it my mission to write this book. A book that would allow me to cook the way I have always cooked: using lovely fresh, vibrant and colourful ingredients, and interesting cooking methods while providing something different for my whole family to enjoy.

I wanted this book to make it easy for me and my readers to understand what we need to be eating and when, to make sure we are giving our bodies exactly what they need for optimum health both before and during pregnancy.

Healthy eating and eating well is something we should all be thinking about, pregnant or not, and this book will not only help support a healthy pregnancy but also (I hope) encourage you to lead a healthier and more nutritious lifestyle. There is no quick fix for overall good health, but within a few months of eating well-balanced and sensible meals, you will start to notice some fabulous benefits. Your skin and hair will feel better, your energy levels will be up and your digestive health improved. Pregnancy takes its toll on our bodies, so it's essential that we keep the machine well oiled and firing on all cylinders.

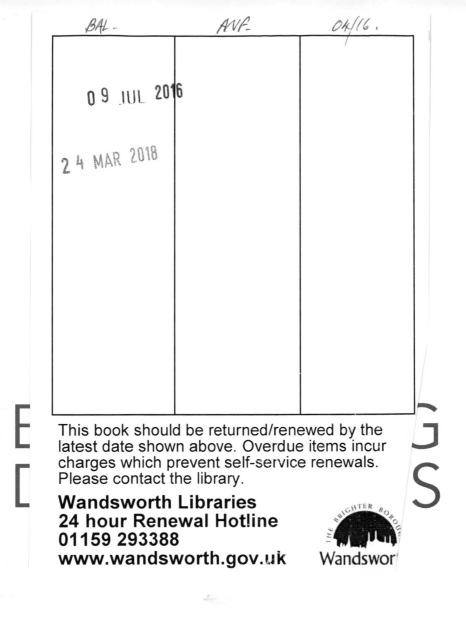

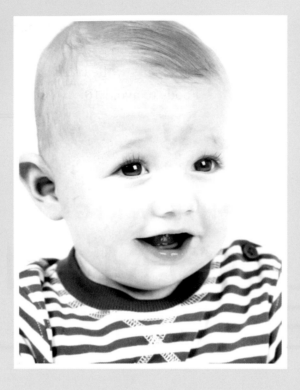

For my beautiful baby boy Albert
Pepper, aka Bertie. Without the
blessing of you, this book would
never have happened. I love you
more than you will ever know.

With that in mind, the recipes in this book are designed to take you through all the stages of your journey. Ideally you should use it from when you first begin trying to conceive right through to when you finally hold your baby and begin the procession of broken nights' sleep.

I know that pregnancy can be tough and at times all you will feel like doing is crawling back to bed with the biscuit tin, but I promise that the recipes in this book are so delicious you honestly won't feel like you are missing out – and there are plenty of sweet treats and snacks to satisfy any cravings!

All pregnant women will need to combat certain ailments at different stages, and I wanted my book to contain recipes that make it easy to cook with certain ingredients, which will hopefully go some way to helping prevent, cure or at least reduce these side effects. In the section 'Food as Medicine' on page 22, we look at common pregnancy ailments, from cramps, constipation and stretch marks, to more serious conditions like anaemia and gestational diabetes. It is packed full of ingredient suggestions and refers to recipes within the book to help assist combat, relieve or, better still, prevent these conditions and the symptoms that most of us assume just come with being pregnant. I am a huge believer that food is nature's medicine and, when used and consumed in the right way, certain foods can make us all feel so much better.

Most importantly, I needed to make sure my recipes were nutritionally balanced and packed full of the right ingredients, so I enlisted the help of nutritional therapist Henrietta Norton (who specialises in pregnancy and preconception). I have been lucky enough to work with Henrietta when I was executive chef at Grace Belgravia, a health and wellbeing club for women in London. She broke down the vitamins and minerals that I needed to include in my diet into a very easy-to-follow nutritional chart (see pages 6–11) and explained where I can find these nutrients and, most importantly, why I needed them. I stuck this chart on to my fridge at home and, with its aid, found menu-planning easy and enjoyable. The recipes that I created using that nutritional chart formed the book you are now reading.

It was so important to me that I should write each recipe and chapter as I experienced it, so the recipes are genuinely what I cooked, ate, blended and juiced while my little one kicked about in my belly.

I truly hope that, wherever you are on your pregnancy journey, this book helps you to feel as well, nourished and inspired by food as you possibly can be. Every woman will have a different pregnancy experience and I have tried my best to take you all into consideration while writing the book. I wish you all well and send all my best for this hugely exciting chapter of your lives. Eat the rainbow, cook with love and enjoy your fabulous journey.

Sophie x

What do you need through your pregnancy and why?

On the following pages, with the help of nutritional therapist Henrietta Norton, I've put together a handy chart showing all the key nutrients, vitamins and minerals you will need while preparing your body for pregnancy, throughout your pregnancy and when/if you breastfeed. Next to every recipe in the book you will see the nutrients as detailed on the chart, helping you to identify them quickly and easily in each dish. This will allow you to plan your weekly meals to ensure that you are getting a well-balanced diet for your baby's optimum growth and development. I found this chart hugely helpful during my pregnancy and I hope you find it as useful and easy to use as I did. The names of the nutrients are written in different-shaped boxes that indicate:

Rectangles	enzymes
Diamonds	minerals, macronutrients and essential fatty acids
Circles	key vitamins

Preconception

WHAT IS IT?	WHY DO I NEED IT?	WHERE CAN I FIND IT?
Coenzyme Q10	Research suggests that an increased intake of coenzyme Q10 can lead to an increased rate of conception.	Sardines, mackerel, pork, beef, chicken, soya bean foods (especially miso and soya beans), spinach, peanuts and sesame seeds.
Iso & Indo-3	Isothiocyanates and indole-3-carbinol help stabilise hormonal balance needed for conception.	Leafy green vegetables, such as bok choi, kale and cabbage, kohlrabi, Brussels sprouts, broccoli and cauliflower.
Phytoestrogens	Thought to moderate conditions associated with hormonal imbalances, such as irregular menstrual cycles, rapid weight gain and loss, excessive or little bleeding during menstruation, which can all affect your ability to ovulate properly.	Soya bean foods (especially miso and soya beans), chickpeas, sprouted seeds (especially alfalfa, mung beans and bean sprouts), lentils and oats.

Preconception, pregnancy and breastfeeding

WHAT IS IT?	WHY DO I NEED IT?	WHERE CAN I FIND IT?
Beta-Caro	Beta-carotene is a form of vitamin A and is needed for a strong immune system. Supports against eye defects in your baby and pre-eclampsia in mums.	Carrots, pumpkin, sweet potato, spinach, broccoli, watercress, tomatoes, peppers, tangerines and apricots.
Calcium	Calcium is vital for making your baby's bones and teeth. It also helps your baby grow a healthy heart, muscles and nerves, and encourages a normal heart rhythm and blood-clotting abilities. If you don't get enough calcium while pregnant, your baby will draw it from your bones, which could lead to osteoporosis in later life. It's import to keep up a good intake of calcium even after you have finished carrying and breastfeeding your baby.	Milk, yogurt, cheese, sardines and fish with soft bones, broccoli, cauliflower and sesame seeds.
Carbs Low GI	Nourishing carbohydrates (low glycaemic index) are great for slow-releasing energy.	Wholegrain and wholemeal bread, brown rice, wholemeal pasta, pulses, carrots, beetroot, squash and most other root vegetables.
Choline	Needed for the delivery of fatty acids and synthesis of membranes in baby's nervous system.	Eggs, fish, soya bean foods (especially miso and soya beans), peanuts and wholegrains.
Fibre	Roughage helps move food through the digestive system and keeps our guts healthy and happy. It prevents constipation and allows for maximum absorption of vital nutrients, which will pass to your baby through the placenta.	Wholegrains, nuts, seeds, fruits and vegetables.
	Soluble fibre helps stabilise blood sugar.	Oats, fruits, vegetables and lentils.

WHAT IS IT?	WHY DO I NEED IT?	WHERE CAN I FIND IT?
Folate	Folate (vitamin B9) is recommended by NICE and the NHS. Their suggested dosage is 400 micrograms (mcg) while trying to conceive and until you are 12 weeks pregnant, to reduce the risk of neural tube defects including spina bifida. It is also important to maintain healthy levels of folate in your diet while pregnant to prevent the risk of folate-deficiency anaemia, which can lead to mum feeling nauseous, faint and tired. Research has also shown that good levels of folate can reduce the risk of your baby being born with a cleft palate and/or cleft lip. Folate works with vitamin B12 to form healthy red blood cells. High levels can also help improve Apgar scores at birth. This is a test carried out by a midwife immediately after the baby's birth, to check Activity, Pulse, Grimace, Appearance and Respiration.	Pulses (especially lentils, adzuki beans, chickpeas and black-eyed beans), kale, spinach, peanuts, Brussels sprouts, asparagus, sesame seeds, broccoli and yeast extract such as Marmite. Folate is easily destroyed by cooking, so these vegetables are best eaten raw or al dente when possible.
Gingerols	Helps to prevent morning sickness.	Ginger.
Iodine	Important for the development of a healthy nervous system, especially during the first three months of pregnancy.	Seafood, eggs, dairy products, shitake mushrooms and seaweed.
Iron	Good iron levels are essential throughout pregnancy and while breastfeeding to avoid anaemia, which can lead to you feeling tired, fatigued and faint. Iron is essential for healthy red blood cells, which carry oxygen around your body as well as to the placenta, which feeds the baby. Low iron levels have been connected with premature babies and babies of low birth weight. Calcium stops your body absorbing iron, so try to avoid mixing iron and calcium in the same sitting.	Present in most red meats but also in chicken, dark leafy green vegetables, beetroot, dried fruit, baked beans, lentils, nuts and seeds.
Magnesium	Deficiency in magnesium is associated with infertility and possible increase of miscarriage. It is also vital for obtaining the full benefits of calcium to form bone, proteins and fatty acids. Thought of as nature's tranquilliser, it helps to relax muscles and reduce stress and anxiety during pregnancy.	Leafy green vegetables, wheatgerm, buckwheat, bananas, almonds, cashews, Brazil nuts, pulses (especially lentils, chickpeas and black-eyed beans), quinoa, pumpkin seeds, sunflower seeds and sprouted seeds (especially alfalfa, mung beans and bean sprouts).

WHAT IS IT?	WHY DO I NEED IT?	WHERE CAN I FIND IT?
Manganese	Manganese helps protect cells from damage, helps form bones and cartilage, and boosts energy levels. It is the second most important mineral after potassium, and low levels of manganese have been linked with defective ovulation.	Watercress, pineapple, okra, endive, blackberries, raspberries, leafy green vegetables and oats.
Omega-3	Omega-3 (DHA or docosahexaenoic acid) is needed for the absorption of vitamins A, D, E and K, and is also a primary structural component of the human brain. Omega-3 and other fatty acids are thought to be beneficial in preparation for pregnancy.	Salmon, mackerel, sardines, tuna, trout, leafy green vegetables, nuts, seeds and rapeseed and flaxseed oil.
Omega-6	Believed to be beneficial to the eye and brain development of infants, and to reduce the risk of low birth weight.	Sunflower oil, pumpkin seeds, sesame seeds and sunflower seeds.
Potassium	Needed for maintaining electrolyte and fluid balance in your body's cells. Potassium also helps the muscles to contract, which is necessary during labour.	Pulses, dried fruits, almonds, cashews, Brazil nuts and wheatgerm.
Selenium	An antioxidant which protects primarily against cell damage and helps support the immune system. Evidence has shown that a good intake of selenium combined with iron during pregnancy can lead to babies having a reduced risk of developing eczema and asthma.	Brazil nuts, tuna, lentils, white fish such as cod, haddock and hake, lamb, turkey, chicken, avocados and shellfish.
Vit A	Vitamin A is needed to maintain good general health and supports a strong immune system, good vision and reproduction. It is especially important when breastfeeding for baby's eyes and skin, and to support your baby's immune system. However, too much can be dangerous, so you don't need to seek it out in the foods you eat. Beta-carotene is converted by the body into vitamin A, so if you are following a healthy diet, you will get all that you need.	Cheese, whole milk, eggs, oily fish, fruits and vegetables, especially broccoli.
Vit B2	Vitamin B2 (riboflavin) is an essential vitamin which helps your body produce energy. It is needed for the growth of healthy skin and good vision, and is essential for baby's eye, bone, muscle and nerve development.	Milk, yogurt, breakfast cereals, wholegrains, almonds, soya bean foods (especially miso and soya beans), mushrooms, spinach and yeast extract such as Marmite.

Vit B6

Vitamin B6 helps your body process proteins, fats and carbohydrates. It also helps form red blood cells and essential antibodies, and is very important for your baby's brain development. Some research shows that a little extra vitamin B6 in our diet can reduce the symptoms of morning sickness. Deficiency could lead to inability to conceive or miscarriage.

Salmon, tuna, turkey, chicken, sweet potatoes, wholegrains, sunflower seeds, hazelnuts, walnuts, peanuts, bananas and avocados.

Vit B12

Vitamin B12 is needed in order for the body to process folate and it helps to protect against anaemia. It also releases energy from foods. It is needed for your baby to produce healthy red blood cells, a healthy nervous system and for general good development.

Found in most foods of animal origin, such as beef, chicken, pork, fish, dairy products and eggs. Also present in soya products and yeast extracts such as Marmite.

Vit C

Vitamin C protects your body's cells and keeps them healthy. Essential for making collagen, which in turn helps make cartilage, tendons, bones and skin, and helps with muscle repair and growth. Also increases the absorption of iron, and is thought to help strengthen capillaries, which can reduce the chance of heavy bleeding. Additionally, vitamin C is an antioxidant, which has been shown to reduce the risk of DNA damage to the ovum and sperm.

Strawberries, oranges, kiwi fruit, tomatoes, sweet potatoes, peppers, peas, leafy green vegetables, broccoli and cauliflower. Fruit and vegetables containing vitamin C are best eaten raw to ensure maximum intake.

Vit D

We get most of our vitamin D needs from the sun, however it is recommend by the NHS that pregnant women take 10 micrograms of vitamin D while pregnant and breastfeeding. This helps with the absorption of calcium, required to form and grow healthy bones in your baby, and is particularly important during the later stages of pregnancy and while breastfeeding. Lack of vitamin D can lead to bone deficiency and weak bones (rickets is a disease that is linked with vitamin D deficiency). It is essential for healthy immune development in baby and promoting immune defences.

Eggs, cottage cheese, oily fish.

WHAT IS IT?	WHY DO I NEED IT?	WHERE CAN I FIND IT?
Vit E	Vitamin E helps maintain cell structure by protecting cell membranes. Studies have suggested, as reported by Allergy UK, that a mother's diet lacking vitamin E could result in the increased risk of children from birth to five years developing asthma. Vitamin E will also help reduce the risk of stretch marks and scarring.	Found in most fresh fruits and vegetables such as broccoli, tomatoes, peas and carrots, as well as hazelnuts, seed oils and oily fish.
Vit K	Vitamin K plays a vital role in the good development of baby's bones and it also helps with clotting, resulting in less bleeding after the birth. Vitamin K can only be absorbed by eating foods that are rich in it. Our bodies do not produce it, which is why a vitamin K injection will routinely be given to your baby immediately after birth. This will reduce the risk of possible internal bleeding in baby before it has had a chance to build up its own supply.	Leafy green vegetables, peas, red cabbage, artichokes, asparagus, celery, rhubarb, rapeseed oil and dairy products.
Zinc	Zinc helps our bodies to produce new cells and enzymes, which grow rapidly during pregnancy. It also helps support our immune system, improves sense of taste and helps with the healing process. Essentially zinc helps our bodies process fats, proteins and carbohydrates. Zinc deficiency studies have shown a link to miscarriage and babies of low birth weight.	Most meat and dairy products, wholegrains, wholewheat bread and pasta, lentils, sprouts (especially alfalfa, mung beans and bean sprouts), seeds and nuts.

Understanding your food groups

This section will help you gain a better understanding of the food groups I have briefly referred to in the nutritional table (see pages 6–11). I hope that these explanations will give you the basic understanding you require as to why we need specific foods at specific times.

Protein

Protein provides amino acids, the building blocks of human tissue, so is vital for the growth of your placenta and your baby during pregnancy. It supports the big changes that happen to our bodies when we are pregnant, and is also needed for the production of breast milk once the baby is born.

Healthy sources of protein are chicken and fish, eggs and dairy products such as yogurt. Pulses such as baked beans, chickpeas and kidney beans, quinoa and even wholemeal bread are good sources of protein too. If you are vegetarian or vegan, mixing your intake of pulses with salads, vegetable stews and vegetable soups is the best way to ensure a full mix of the amino acids needed for growth.

Carbohydrates

Carbohydrates come in two forms, which I like to refer to as: 'nourishing' and 'less-nourishing'.

NOURISHING CARBOHYDRATES are slow-releasing energy foods or those with a low glycaemic index (GI). These foods are broken down slowly in our bodies, leading to a gradual increase in blood sugar and energy, so we feel fuller for longer. Nourishing carbohydrates can be found in pulses, wholegrains such as barley, spelt and porridge oats, and some less sweet fruits and vegetables.

LESS-NOURISHING CARBOHYDRATES or those with a high GI are high in sugar and break down very quickly in our bodies, causing our blood-sugar levels to spike. This can cause sugar highs and crashes, leave you feeling unsatisfied, and can lead to excess weight gain. Foods containing less-nourishing carbohydrates like cakes, biscuits, white bread and highly processed foods in general, should be eaten in moderation.

Carbohydrates are the main source of energy in our diet and are important during pregnancy. They also provide an array of nutrients, including magnesium and B vitamins, which are needed for your baby too. These can be found in foods such as pulses, wholegrains, sugar-free breakfast cereals, oats and various fruits and vegetables such as new potatoes, sweet potatoes, apricots and less-ripe bananas. They are essential for baby's eye, bone, nerve and muscle development, as well as helping your body to process that essential folate.

There is no need to increase your carbohydrate intake specifically during pregnancy, but remember that, for general health, nourishing carbohydrates should make up 50 per cent of your diet. This doesn't just mean grains: vegetables such as parsnips, carrots, potatoes, butternut squash and other roots are also sources of carbohydrates.

Fibre

There are two types of fibre. The first is insoluble fibre, found in breakfast cereals such as bran, and wholemeal bread, which helps to move roughage along the digestive tract and prevents constipation. The second type is soluble fibre, found in oats, fruits, vegetables and lentils, which is needed to help stabilise blood-sugar levels and therefore energy levels.

Fats

Despite their bad name, dietary fats are crucial for good health. They play a vital role in the body, making cell membranes for your baby and ensuring nerve health and development. They are also used to 'ferry' fat-soluble nutrients to your baby, such as vitamins A, E and K. Some fats are healthier than others, though, and it is important to understand the different types.

Pregnancy is a time in our life when fats become even more essential in our diet, especially the type of fat called 'essential fatty acids'.

The healthy fats:

POLYUNSATURATED FATS

These healthy fats provide the building blocks for making the membranes found in body cells, including the heart muscle cells, brain cells and arteries for your baby.

Omega-3 fatty acids, one of the specialised fats known as essential fatty acids (the other being omega-6 fatty acids), belong to this group of polyunsaturated fats. These fats are especially important for a healthy brain for you and your baby, particularly during the first and third trimester, when rapid brain and nervous system development is occurring.

Your omega-3 stores will be going to your baby. Insufficient intake of these fats has also been linked to increased risk of atopic allergies such as eczema in children. Good sources of omega-3 include mackerel, herring, salmon, trout, sardines, pilchards, fresh tuna, wild game such as venison, omega-3-enriched eggs and walnuts.

MONOUNSATURATED FATS

These are healthy fats and they should be eaten as part of a healthy and balanced diet. Foods that are rich in monounsaturated fats include avocados, peanuts, cashews, almonds, sunflower seeds and plant-based cooking oils such as rapeseed and sunflower oil.

You will see that I have used mainly rapeseed oil, extra virgin olive oil and avocado oil throughout this book to help you fulfil your healthy fat quota, all of which can be bought in supermarkets or health-food shops.

Nuts and seeds are an essential part of our daily balanced diet, as they contain huge amounts of minerals that contribute to a healthy lifestyle and pregnancy. They are also an excellent source of protein. Nut allergies are often a worry during pregnancy because of previous advice to not eat them for fear of causing an allergic reaction. This advice has now been changed and the NHS only recommends avoiding nuts if you have previously had a reaction to them. Nuts make a brilliant snack and can nourish you with lots of essential vitamins and minerals such as vitamin E, folate, magnesium, manganese and omega-6, all of which will contribute to your health and that of your baby.

The healthy fats but in moderation:
SATURATED FATS

Saturated fats have gained a bit of a bad reputation because consuming them in excess has been associated with an increased risk of coronary heart disease and excessive weight gain. However, this is not the case if eaten in moderation (small amounts of butter or whole milk, or eating the fat in your meat). A small amount of saturated fat is needed and should be enjoyed as part of a healthy diet. Saturated fats are needed to produce important hormones in our body during pregnancy. However, we do not need too much saturated fat so it's best to base your fat intake on the other healthy fats instead.

Sources of saturated fat include dairy products such as butter and cheese, and red meat.

The non-healthy fats:
TRANS FATS

Trans fats are the result of hydrogenated, processed or refined oils and they are found in processed foods such as mass-produced cakes, biscuits and margarines. The body processes trans fats in a way that is harmful to health. They can stop you from being able to use essential fatty acids (see page 13) in foods and pass them to your baby, can cause blood sugar irregularity (causing energy slumps and brain fog) and promote weight gain. Always check labels for trans fats or partially hydrogenated fats.

Preserving nutrients while cooking

Some people believe that raw food is better for us than cooked. This isn't strictly true, as sometimes the cooking process can disarm harmful enzymes (for example, in beans and pulses) and foods such as poultry need to be heated above 80°C (175°F) to destroy any dangerous bacteria.

However, vitamins and nutrients can be destroyed by overcooking, so eating your vegetables raw or al dente is a good way to ensure you get their maximum nutritional value. Steaming rather than boiling, or grilling rather than frying is a good way of maintaining vitamins in foods.

Minerals, however, are not destroyed by heat. Cooked or raw, food will still contain the same amounts of calcium, magnesium, iron, zinc and manganese, to name but a few. The only exception is potassium, which escapes into the cooking liquid as food cooks.

The recipes in this book use a range of cooking methods to ensure a good balance of healthy preparation while ensuring maximum flavour in your meals.

Foods to avoid

The NHS has very clear guidelines regarding which foods should be avoided during pregnancy. These guidelines are in place as certain foods are more likely to cause food poisoning which could potentially harm your baby.

RAW OR UNDERCOOKED MEAT carries a potential risk of toxoplasmosis, an infection caused by a parasite. It can also be found in soil, untreated water and cat faeces. This can be highly dangerous to your unborn baby, though cases are rare. Cook your meat thoroughly and ensure that no traces of blood or pinkness are present, especially in pork, chicken, sausages, red meat and burgers.

PÂTÉS, including those made with liver, meat, fish and vegetables, are not considered safe as they may carry listeria bacteria, which causes food poisoning.

LIVER contains high levels of vitamin A, excessive amounts of which may be harmful to your unborn baby.

CURED MEATS such as salami, chorizo and Parma ham have not been cooked and therefore could contain the parasite that causes toxoplasmosis. If eaten on a pizza or in a stew which has been heated above 80°C (175°F), however, they are considered safe.

SWORDFISH, SHARK AND MARLIN should be avoided due to their high mercury content, and tuna should be eaten in moderation. Try not to exceed 280g fresh tuna or 560g drained tinned tuna per week.

SHELLFISH such as crab, lobster, prawns, mussels, clams and scallops are all considered safe if very fresh and thoroughly cooked. Raw shellfish can contain bacteria, which may cause food poisoning.

CHEESE is a good source of calcium but you do need to be a bit careful what cheeses you eat when pregnant. Soft mould-ripened cheeses, such as soft cheese with a white rind (e.g. Brie, Camembert and chèvre) and soft blue-veined cheese (e.g. Roquefort, Danish blue and Gorgonzola) provide a favourable environment for bacteria (such as listeria) to grow. However, they are considered safe if cooked thoroughly. Soft unpasteurised cheeses should be avoided for similar reasons. Make sure any soft cheeses (such as mozzarella, feta and cottage cheese), which aren't mould-ripened, are pasteurised and they are considered safe to eat both uncooked or cooked. Most hard cheeses, even if they are unpasteurised, are considered safe to eat cooked or uncooked, as they don't have the moist environment for bacteria to grow in like soft cheeses do. If you are unsure, the NHS website lists many common cheeses that are considered safe and unsafe to eat when pregnant.

UNPASTEURISED MILK AND YOGURT contain bacteria and should not be eaten or drunk during pregnancy.

RAW OR PARTIALLY COOKED EGGS may contain salmonella. Although this is unlikely to cause harm to your baby it can cause vomiting and diarrhoea in the mother, which can lead to dehydration and require medical attention.

FISH OIL SUPPLEMENTS and other supplements high in vitamin A, which may be harmful to your unborn baby.

ALL FOODS GROWN IN THE SOIL should be washed thoroughly to remove any harmful bacteria.

NUTS: if you have nut allergies or if allergies run in the family, the NHS advises not eating nuts while pregnant. If not, eating nuts is encouraged to build up your baby's tolerance.

HERBAL AND GREEN TEAS: the Food Standards Agency advises drinking no more than two cups per day during pregnancy. Many herbal teas, and especially green teas, contain caffeine which isn't recommended while pregnant. We know very little about the true effects of drinking herbal teas while pregnant so it is best to err on the side of caution. Try fresh mint tea or fresh ginger-infused water instead.

Supplements

Some women have had marginally sufficient levels of nutrients in order to 'tick over' throughout their life so far. However, during pregnancy, this marginal status is not enough to supply both them and their baby and they can find themselves feeling very tired, experiencing unwanted pregnancy symptoms such as digestive issues, or succumbing easily to colds and flu. In addition, many women find it hard to eat as well as they would like in the early stages because of morning sickness.

The NHS recommends that all pregnant women take 400mcg of folic acid daily before conception and during the first 12 weeks of pregnancy, and 10mcg of vitamin D daily for the entire pregnancy. Iron supplements can be beneficial if you test positive for iron-deficiency anaemia, and omega-3 supplements are a good way of ensuring you are getting enough DHA (see the nutritional chart on page 9). There is a some evidence to suggest that vitamin B6 supplements can reduce nausea and vomiting in pregnancy too.

However, this is the base minimum, and many experts recommend taking a good multivitamin and mineral supplement formulated specifically for pregnancy, and for breastfeeding.

If you are on medication, check with your GP before taking any supplements.

Vegetarians and vegans

Although this book is not aimed directly at vegetarians and vegans, I am confident that with a few small tweaks the recipes can be adapted to ensure a balanced diet for all, whatever your lifestyle and dietary choices. If you do follow a vegetarian or vegan diet, you may find it harder to access some of the required nutrients during pregnancy, especially iron and vitamin B12. To make sure your diet is rich in iron, eat plenty of pulses, wholemeal bread, dark leafy vegetables, dried fruits such as apricots, breakfast cereals with added iron, and eggs if your diet allows them. You can also help your body to absorb iron by upping your intake of vitamin C after an iron-heavy meal. You could, for example, drink a glass of fresh orange juice after eating a meal containing spinach and eggs. Calcium prevents iron being absorbed, so if you are trying to increase your iron intake, avoid mixing iron-rich foods and calcium-rich foods. Have these at different times of the day. For example, try having baked beans on seeded toast for breakfast, followed by some fresh fruit and a glass of juice; a spinach and watercress salad with roasted tomatoes and lentils for lunch; and macaroni cheese followed by a yogurt for dinner.

You can get B12 from cheese, milk, eggs, soya bean products, fortified breakfast cereals and yeast extract such as Marmite. You can also get your much-needed protein from many different sources, including eggs, cottage cheese, quinoa, pulses, peanut butter, yogurt, nuts and tofu.

If you are vegan, your calcium intake needs to be increased while pregnant, especially during the third trimester and while breastfeeding (if choosing to do so). This will help the baby form strong bones and teeth, and helps protect you against osteoporosis in later life. You can get added calcium from fortified soya, rice and oat drinks. Calcium is also found in sources such as tofu, tahini and sesame seed pastes, dark leafy vegetables, pulses and dried fruit.

Sugar

Pregnant women often have cravings for sugar and find it hard to resist. Excess sugar can lead to unwanted weight gain, which can sometimes be hard to shift after the baby is born. Unfortunately, sugar is hidden in so much of the food we eat today that even those of us without a sweet tooth may be consuming more than we should. Sugar is a carbohydrate which naturally occurs in milk, fruit, honey, maple syrup and root vegetables, to name but a few, in the forms of lactose, glucose and fructose. Sugar can cause our blood-sugar levels to peak, giving us that temporary high followed by a rather nasty sugar crash, which in turn can leave us feeling tired, grumpy and craving more sugar.

It's not all bad news, though, as our bodies need a certain amount of sugar in order to send energy to our muscles and keep our brains active. During pregnancy our bodies are using huge amounts of energy to support our growing babies and changing bodies, so a little sugar is necessary. The best forms of sugar to use (as found in the recipes in this book) are the following:

Manuka honey

Found in large supermarkets and health-food shops, active manuka honey from New Zealand will carry the UMF trademark and a number from 5+ up to 45+. The higher the number, the more active and expensive the honey will be. If you are using manuka honey to cook with, a lower number is more than acceptable. Methylglyoxal, a compound with the capacity to kill bacteria and viruses, is found in most types of honey but is highest in manuka. Manuka honey is also said to have anti-inflammatory qualities, to counteract nausea and acid indigestion, and can help predigest starchy foods such as bread.

If manuka honey is out of your price range, try to get the next best thing, i.e. a honey that isn't mass-produced and highly processed. A good quality jar of honey will usually be around the £5–£8 mark. Raw manuka and raw honey is also available, and is considered to have excellent health qualities; however, it is not recommend that pregnant women eat raw honey, as it is completely unpasteurised and may contain bacteria that could be considered harmful.

Maple syrup and agave nectar

These are two sugar substitutes that, although not strictly considered to be good for us, are natural products and therefore contain some natural traces of minerals not found in refined sugar. They are, however, high in glucose (maple syrup) and fructose (agave nectar), which cause blood sugar spikes, and so should be consumed in moderation.

Gluten and wheat intolerance

More and more people these days suffer with an intolerance or allergy to gluten and wheat. Gluten is present in so many of the foods we eat and is often hard to avoid in processed food and baked goods, unless you cook them yourself from scratch. I have tried throughout this book to give alternatives to wheat and gluten, in the form brown rice flour, buckwheat flour and chickpea flour.

I find these three flours work well in a whole host of recipes where wheat flour is usually present. If you have never suffered from a gluten or wheat intolerance, it is unlikely you will while pregnant and there is no reason to avoid them. Excessive gluten in the diet has been linked with constipation, however, which can be more of a problem during pregnancy. If you are suffering with this, try reducing your gluten intake and upping your fibre in the form of fresh fruit and vegetables, brown rice, bulgur wheat, quinoa and buckwheat.

Dairy and lactose intolerances

There are many non-dairy alternatives widely available, lots of which are truly delicious and nutritionally beneficial, and I have tried to give alternatives to dairy where possible throughout the book. Unsweetened almond and hazelnut milks are among my favourite ingredients, so you will see these popping up often. Unsweetened soya milk is also a good alternative to cows' milk, should you have an intolerance or fancy an alternative. If you don't have a problem with lactose it's a good idea to keep up your intake of dairy products throughout pregnancy, as it is a very quick and easy way of consuming much-needed calcium. You can substitute the milks in most of the recipes in this book, so feel free to use your favourite.

Eating organic?

In an ideal world, all the food we buy and eat would be organic and therefore free from herbicides and pesticides. Although the chemicals that are used to grow and rear the foods we eat are not considered harmful to humans, there have been very few studies and tests carried out to reveal what effects a cocktail of these chemicals may have on our health.

Every year Pesticides Action Network UK publishes its list of the fruits and vegetables that are most likely to have been exposed to herbicides and pesticides, and therefore these are the ones that you may want to consider buying organic. At the time of writing the list is (from most affected): citrus fruits, pineapples, pears, apples, grapes, strawberries, nectarines and peaches, tomatoes, apricots, parsnips, cucumbers, carrots. Lettuce, peas and beans in pods, sweet potatoes and courgettes are also on the list of foods containing high levels of pesticide residue.

Others foods considered to have high pesticide residue and which you may want to buy organic are oily fish, cereal grains, flour and dried fruits.

With regard to meat, if you can afford to buy organic and grass-fed then this is the best option in terms of reducing the number of chemicals you are exposed to. Not only this, but you will also have peace of mind knowing that the food you are eating has been reared and farmed using sustainable and ethical farming methods.

If you are struggling to source organic foods in your local supermarket, try shopping at your local farmers' markets or perhaps look into signing up to an organic food box delivery service.

Of course not everyone can afford to buy organic food and please rest assured that by eating a healthy and balanced diet you and your baby will be perfectly well nourished.

Food as medicine

There are huge amounts of advice and traditional food-related remedies available to women suffering with common pregnancy ailments. Some of these are tried and tested, and have been proven to work; others are a little more hit and miss, working for some women but not for others. Ultimately, all pregnancies are different and your own experiences will be unique to you and your body.

During pregnancy, we are limited as to what medication we can take and many of us try not to take any medication at all (always check with your doctor or midwife before taking any medicines while pregnant). However, some foods have known medicinal properties that may just help to relieve you of a certain symptom and give you a little respite from whatever is causing the discomfort.

Most importantly, having a well-balanced diet throughout your pregnancy should help you to feel in good shape to support yourself and your growing baby for the next nine months, as well as during the early months of parenthood.

Over the next few pages are some of the most common complaints experienced during each of the trimesters and some ways you can help combat them or ease your symptoms through the foods you eat.

Common in the first trimester

Headaches and dizziness

Headaches and dizziness are common complaints for lots of expectant mums in their first trimester; however, you can experience them at any stage of pregnancy. If you are suffering, try to:

KEEP UP YOUR INTAKE OF VITAMIN C by eating strawberries, apples, tomatoes and oranges, which all contain high levels of vitamin C.

STAY WELL HYDRATED by drinking 2–3 litres of water per day. Water can also help with morning sickness as small sips can help counter the feeling of nausea. Its also important to replace any lost fluids.

EAT LITTLE AND OFTEN to help control blood-sugar levels. Peaks and dips can cause light-headedness and headaches. Small healthy snacks are good to have to hand (see the chapter on Healthy Snacks, page 168).

KEEP UP LEVELS OF VITAMIN E AND IRON as these help to control circulation and can prevent you from feeling faint. Try healthy snacks such as almonds and seeds (see my recipe for Sweet and Salty Munchy Seeds and Nuts on page 176). All leafy green vegetables such as kale, spinach and broccoli are high in iron, as well as lean red meat such as steak.

RECOMMENDED RECIPES: Broccoli, Almond, Chilli and Lemon Wholewheat Fusilli (page 75); Spinach, Kale and Watercress Soup (page 161).

Morning sickness

Morning sickness is extremely common and usually occurs during weeks 6–12, though some women suffer from it throughout their pregnancy. It is thought to be due to hormonal changes, but has also been linked to a lack of vitamin B6 in a woman's diet. The remedies below are not fail-safe: some women swear by them and others seem to think they have no effect at all! They are all worth a try, however, if it goes some way to making you feel a little better.

NOURISHING CARBOHYDRATES, slow-releasing energy foods such as brown rice and wholemeal bread and pasta will help you feel fuller for longer and stabilise your blood-sugar levels, which may keep nausea at bay.

GINGER is well known for its anti-sickness properties. Historically, ginger has a long tradition of being very effective in alleviating symptoms of gastrointestinal distress. In herbal medicine ginger is regarded as an excellent 'carminative' (a substance which promotes the elimination of intestinal gas) and it is used to relax and soothe the intestinal tract. Try some fresh ginger grated into sparkling water or some ginger cordial, and add fresh ginger to food whenever you can or simply sip a cold ginger ale.

FENNEL, either fresh or fennel seeds, has often been used to ward off nausea. Fennel has long been used as a digestive aid to soothe bloating, heartburn and an upset stomach.

It works by relaxing and easing muscle spasms in the gastrointestinal tract, which in turn calms symptoms such as cramping and gas. Try some fennel tea, or make your own by crushing some seeds in warm boiled water. Raw fennel thinly sliced and served as a salad with a squeeze of lemon juice on top is refreshing and delicious.

SOUR FRUITS can be used to excite your bored and changing taste buds, and distract you from feeling sick. Increased levels of oestrogen and progesterone are thought to play a role in the changes to our taste buds during early pregnancy, causing us to suddenly go off food we once loved. The medical term 'dysgeusia', meaning an altered sense of taste, accounts for this difference in perception. Try crisp green apples, lemons, limes and grapefruit.

FRESH MINT AND PEPPERMINT, like ginger, is one of the most well-known remedies to help ward off sickness and tummy troubles. Some women like to put a few drops of peppermint oil into a glass of water as it helps soothe the digestive tract, and others prefer to inhale a little of the vapour as the menthol quality relieves the feeling of sickness. Fresh mint infused into warm water or cold sparking water with a spritz of lemon or lime is a good thirst-quenching drink that may help keep sickness at bay. Peppermint sweets or chewing gum may also help with the sickness.

RECOMMENDED RECIPES: Poached Chicken with Ginger and Lemongrass Broth (page 80); Fennel and Flaxseed Oatcakes (page 175).

Tiredness

Tiredness is very common throughout pregnancy and it's nothing to worry about. Remember that your body is working hard to ensure that your baby is well nourished and growing as he or she should. Try to follow the advice below to help counteract it a little.

STAY WELL HYDRATED as plenty of water is essential for a healthy digestive system, which my become sluggish during pregnancy. It will also allow your body to recover if you suffer from vomiting due to morning sickness.

EAT LITTLE AND OFTEN to control your blood-sugar levels and prevent you feeling light-headed and fatigued.

AVOID FATTY AND SUGARY FOODS, especially before bedtime, as these can play havoc with blood-sugar and energy levels.

INCREASE YOUR INTAKE OF NOURISHING CARBOHYDRATES as the slow-releasing energy will help you feel more balanced and help prevent energy highs and lows.

EAT MORE PROTEIN as not eating enough can contribute to tiredness. Aim to eat a source of protein with each meal to stabilise blood sugar fluctuations.

TAKE NAPS if you are tired. Your body is working overtime so make sure to take breaks, have little power naps at the weekend and, if you are lucky enough, sit down during your commute to work. Relax when you can.

RECOMMENDED RECIPES: Hearty Lamb and Root Vegetable Stew with Barley (page 87); Healthy Chicken and Sweet Potato Chips (page 82).

Common in the second and third trimesters

Anaemia

This is quite common in pregnancy, especially around the 20-week mark when your body's blood volume rises. Your body doesn't produce more blood; it just dilutes what you already have. Anaemia is a shortage of haemoglobin, which moves oxygen around the body via red blood cells. Lack of haemoglobin can leave you feeling fatigued, dizzy and faint. It can also lead to shortness of breath and headaches and leave you looking rather pale.

KEEP UP YOUR INTAKE OF IRON AND FOLATE, AS WELL AS VITAMIN B12 by eating a good, varied and well-balanced diet. These minerals and vitamins can be found in spinach, kale, wholegrains, pulses and beans, dried fruits such as apricots, and lean meat such as turkey.

VITAMIN C HELPS YOUR BODY ABSORB IRON, so keep up your intake of fresh fruits and vegetables such as strawberries, oranges, tomatoes, kiwi fruit, peas and broccoli. Don't overcook your vegetables, as vitamin C is easily destroyed; instead, eat them raw or very lightly steamed, for maximum nutritional value. Try drinking a glass of orange or tomato juice after eating an iron-rich meal to help absorption.

AVOID EATING CALCIUM WITH IRON because calcium prevents the body's absorption of iron. Calcium is needed for your baby's bone development among other things so try to eat foods containing these two minerals at different times. For example, try having Steak, Tomato and Roasted Red Onion Salad (page 107) for lunch and drink a glass of fresh orange juice or a green high-iron juice from the Juices, Smoothies, Teas and Warming Drinks chapter (page 204) just after your main meal to help you absorb the iron.

RECOMMENDED RECIPES: Steak, Tomato and Roasted Red Onion Salad (page 107); Blackened Fish with Guacamole and Black-eyed Bean Tacos (page 104); Folate Lift juice (page 208).

Constipation

You may find that during pregnancy you become constipated. In the early stages, this is due to the hormone progesterone slowing down your digestive system; then, increasingly, as your pregnancy progresses and you get closer to your due date, it is because there is a rather large baby sitting on your large intestine, making things sluggish. It can be very uncomfortable and leave you feeling slow, heavy and bloated. It can also cause cramps, stomach ache and a loss of appetite. Iron supplements can also bring on a bout of constipation. Symptoms can be greatly improved by making small changes to your diet; however, if you are still suffering after trying the recommendations below, talk to your midwife, who may be able to prescribe a natural laxative.

KEEP UP FLUID INTAKE by drinking 10 glasses of water a day. A glass of warm water with the juice of half a lemon in the morning can help kick-start your digestive system.

KEEP UP YOUR FIBRE INTAKE, especially from plenty of raw fruits and vegetables. Prunes and prune juice are particularly good for relieving symptoms of constipation.

REGULAR, GENTLE EXERCISE like swimming (although avoid breaststroke as it can cause problems with your hips during pregnancy, especially in the third trimester), pregnancy yoga and Pilates, and walking can all help keep things moving. Try to walk for 20–30 minutes every day to keep active.

EAT LITTLE AND OFTEN as overeating can put a strain on your stomach and therefore your digestive system, making it hard to process food. Make sure you chew your food properly.

EAT PLENTY OF ESSENTIAL FATTY ACIDS because these are really important for maintaining a regular digestive system. Avocados, salmon, mackerel and flaxseed oil can all help lubricate the bowel.

PRUNES, DRIED FRUITS, NUTS AND WHOLEGRAINS can all help, but watch that these don't contribute to the problem and bulk things up. Try adding more fibre slowly (a few prunes on your yogurt for breakfast) at first, to see if it's helping or hindering things.

MAGNESIUM is needed for peristaltic movement in the gut, the movement that pushes food through to the bowel. Eat foods high in magnesium, such as seeds and green leafy vegetables, to help ensure everything is functioning as it should. You could also consider a magnesium supplement, but seek advice from a professional before doing so and check that your pregnancy supplement doesn't already give you a dose.

RECOMMENDED RECIPES: Earl Grey and Ginger Prune Compote (page 95); Quinoa Bircher with Natural Yogurt and Stewed Plums (page 96); Breakfast on the Go smoothie (page 209); Asian Salmon Lettuce Cups (page 121).

Gestational diabetes

This can sometimes be diagnosed in the third trimester of pregnancy, with most women being checked for it by a routine blood test at 28 weeks. Gestational diabetes is a condition caused by your cells becoming more resistant to insulin during pregnancy. It is usually temporary and will disappear once the baby arrives. For some women this condition is unavoidable, but there are many ways in which doctors and midwives can treat, control and monitor it. However, there are a few things you can do to reduce your risk of developing gestational diabetes.

If you have a family history of diabetes, are overweight or have had gestational diabetes with a previous pregnancy, you will be at greater risk, so please keep an eye out for the signs, which include feeling faint, dizziness and severe tiredness, and make sure to visit your midwife regularly.

LIMIT YOUR INTAKE OF PROCESSED SUGAR, which can cause our body's glucose levels to spike and trigger excessive insulin production, which can in turn lead to diabetes. Keep your consumption of cakes, biscuits and fizzy drinks down.

TRY TO AVOID EATING TOO MUCH FRUIT and make sure that your five-a-day is balanced with both fruit and vegetables. Fruit, although good for us as it contains vitamins, minerals, water and antioxidants, still contains fruit sugar called fructose.

The benefits of eating fruit when you need a sugar hit rather than eating sweets or cakes is that fruit contains fibre, which slows down the body's digestion of glucose, preventing the extreme sugar peaks and crashes that you get from processed food.

TAKE REGULAR GENTLE EXERCISE 2–3 times a week, for 20–45 minutes. Exercise can help improve glucose tolerance, meaning your body processes and manages insulin and controls blood-sugar levels more effectively. Walking, pregnancy yoga and Pilates, swimming (although avoid breaststroke, especially in the third trimester) and bouncing on a birthing ball are all great.

EAT PLENTY OF NOURISHING, SLOW-RELEASING CARBOHYDRATES THROUGHOUT YOUR PREGNANCY, such as quinoa, brown rice, wholegrains such as spelt, barley and bulgur wheat, and wholemeal bread and pasta. These will help to stabilise your blood sugars and prevent peaks and crashes.

RECOMMENDED RECIPES: Indonesian Rice Pot with Egg and Salmon (page 127); Lamb Cutlets with Saffron, Pistachio and Spinach Rice (page 108); Sumac and Tahini Hummus (page 181).

High blood pressure or hypertension

During the last trimester of your pregnancy, your midwife may ask you about swollen feet, ankles and fingers. This is because she or he is checking for hypertension or signs of pre-eclampsia. Your urine will also be checked for protein. Hypertension can affect your kidney and liver functions and make the heart work harder, and in severe cases it can lead to pre-eclampsia, which, if untreated, could develop into eclampsia, a rare but very serious condition that can restrict blood flow to the unborn baby. The exact cause of pre-eclampsia is not known; however, it is thought to be associated with a problem with the placenta, and can affect up to 5 per cent of pregnancies. If you experience any swelling, please visit your midwife so your blood pressure can be checked. Pre-eclampsia is easily diagnosed and will require a stay in hospital for observation. Thankfully, these conditions can be treated, and you can reduce your chances of developing them by trying to eat a good, wholesome and balanced diet and doing the following:

BE CAREFUL WITH SALT, as excess salt can cause high blood pressure. Use it with care. Try seasoning your food with a spritz of lemon juice when you might otherwise have reached for the salt cellar.

INCLUDE ENOUGH PROTEIN, VITAMIN C AND VITAMIN E, ZINC AND MAGNESIUM IN YOUR DIET because a lack of these can result in hypertension. Be sure to eat plenty of lean meat such as chicken and turkey, fish, tofu, pulses, avocado, and lots of fresh fruit and vegetables, which can help lower your blood pressure.

RECOMMENDED RECIPES: Griddled Buttermilk Chicken with Chickpeas, Sumac and Dates (page 101); Pink Grapefruit, Peach and Pistachio Salad (page 92); Oestrogen Boost juice (page 208).

Hunger

Many women get their appetite back in the second trimester and the urge to eat and satisfy your hunger can sometimes be hard to resist, especially if you haven't felt hungry or interested in food for three months. Hunger during pregnancy is very normal and is often caused by the increase in hormones. Some days you will feel hungrier than others and that's fine and totally normal. Try to keep the idea of a balanced, healthy diet at the back of your mind. Enjoy a treat every now and then and don't be overly strict with yourself. Just be sensible: if you have had a calorie-heavy couple of days, try to eat healthily for the rest of the week.

Try to remember that you don't actually need to consume any extra calories until you are six months pregnant, and then it's only an extra 200 calories per day. Excessive overeating can lead to heartburn, rapid weight gain, stretch marks and even gestational diabetes. Help combat hunger by trying the following:

EAT LITTLE AND OFTEN

KEEP UP FLUID INTAKE by aiming to drink 10 glasses of water a day.

HEALTHY SNACKING can help bridge the gap between mealtimes. Carry healthy, wholesome, fresh and homemade snacks with you when you go out. Fruit, nuts, seeds and oatcakes are all good choices to keep in your bag. See the Healthy Snacks chapter for other ideas (page 168).

AVOID FATTY AND SUGARY FOODS

EAT SLOW-RELEASING ENERGY FOODS to keep you feeling full for longer. (See Nourishing Carbohydrates on page 12.)

RECOMMENDED RECIPES: Apple Chips (page 172); Sesame and Parmesan Kale Crisps (page 174); Peanut Butter, Banana and Oatmeal Cookies (page 191).

Indigestion, reflux and heartburn

A very common complaint all through pregnancy, which unfortunately tends to get worse as your due date gets closer. Reflux and heartburn can be caused by many things but are mainly due to hormonal changes in the first and second trimesters, and then by your growing womb pressing on your stomach in the later stages. As many as 8 in 10 women are thought to suffer with this condition during pregnancy and it can often be very uncomfortable, preventing you from getting a proper night's sleep or eating properly. You can make a few small changes to your diet and lifestyle to relieve the effects of heartburn and indigestion; however, if it's very bad there are remedies available, so talk to your GP or midwife. Antacids are regularly prescribed to pregnant women on the NHS, so don't go and spend a fortune before you've had your midwife appointment. You can also try the following:

EAT LITTLE AND OFTEN

AVOID FATTY, PROCESSED FOODS AND THOSE HIGH IN SUGAR

AVOID ACIDIC FOODS LIKE TOMATOES AND FRUIT JUICES

AVOID CAFFEINE AND FIZZY DRINKS

KEEP UP YOUR FLUID INTAKE IN BETWEEN MEALS – aim to drink about 10 glasses a day.

DON'T EAT TOO LATE OR RIGHT BEFORE BED and allow at least two hours for your food to digest before going to sleep; lying down will increase the symptoms of heartburn and reflux.

TRY DRINKING A GLASS OF COLD MILK BEFORE BED OR WHEN SUFFERING as this may help to neutralise stomach acid.

RECOMMENDED RECIPES: Chicken Kale and Barley Healing Broth (page 165); Pork, Ginger and Buckwheat Soba Noodle Soup (page 166).

Leg cramps

Leg cramps are a very common ailment in pregnancy, especially in the later stages. They are caused by sudden contractions of the muscles, which cause spasm and unpleasant pain. Four out of five women experience this at night, unfortunately, but cramps can usually be sorted out by stretching the calf or affected muscle. You may experience pain or aching after a severe cramp but this shouldn't last for more than a few minutes.

Leg cramps can occur for a variety of reasons. They can be caused by the extra weight you are carrying, or your growing uterus putting extra pressure on the blood supply to your legs, especially in the later stages of pregnancy. Increased pregnancy hormones can also affect the muscle tone in your legs, leading to cramping.

MAKE SURE YOUR INTAKE OF IRON, CALCIUM AND MAGNESIUM IS HIGH ENOUGH. Leg cramps are often caused by a deficiency in these minerals so eat plenty of dark leafy vegetables such as kale, broccoli, spinach and savoy cabbage; dairy products including milk, cheese and natural yogurt; wholegrains such as brown pasta, brown rice, spelt, barley and bulgur wheat; and seeds and nuts.

AVOID SITTING IN ONE POSITION FOR TOO LONG

TAKE REGULAR GENTLE EXERCISE throughout the day: walk to the shops rather than drive, and try swimming (although avoid breaststroke, especially in the third trimester).

STAY REALLY WELL HYDRATED – add a squeeze of lemon or lime to your water to make it a little more interesting.

RECOMMENDED RECIPES: Frozen Greek Yogurt and Pomegranate Cubes (page 196); Beetroot and Hazelnut Dip (page 180); Spelt Eggy Bread with Cottage Cheese and Prune Compote (page 115); Prawn and Artichoke Wholewheat Spaghetti (page 124).

Stretch marks

Stretch marks can occur at any time during or after pregnancy, and can be quite disheartening. They can be caused by a few things, including your bump growing at a rapid rate (as it tends to during the second and third trimester) and your skin stretching too fast. Stretch marks can appear on your breasts, buttocks, stomach, hips and thighs. In some women stretch marks are very common, and if your mother suffered from them the likelihood is that you will as well. You can, however, try a few techniques to stop them becoming too severe and noticeable. Prevention is better than cure in the case of stretch marks, so try incorporating some of the following into your daily routine:

EAT HEALTHILY AND SENSIBLY to avoid rapid weight gain.

MAKE SALMON AND MACKEREL, AVOCADOS, FLAXSEED OIL AND NUTS ESSENTIAL PARTS OF YOUR DIET. Vitamins C and E, zinc and fatty acids help produce collagen and therefore help the skin to become supple. Heal your skin from within.

STAY WELL MOISTURISED by using an oil high in vitamin E (such as sweet almond oil or coconut oil) twice a day on the areas most likely to be affected, concentrating on your breasts, buttocks, belly, hips and thighs. Throughout the book I have cooked with coconut oil, which is a fabulous and flavourful ingredient with many nutritional qualities. These include vitamins E and K, lauric and caprylic acid, and other medium chain fatty acids (MCFA), which all help to restore the protective layers in your skin that may be damaged due to a stretching belly. Organic first-pressed virgin coconut oil is also mild enough to use when breastfeeding and on newborn babies as a moisturiser if you do start to notice dry skin patches or simply want some bonding time with a little baby massage. Coconut oil has antifungal, antibacterial and antioxidant properties, which can also help relieve inflammation and symptoms of eczema.

EXFOLIATE REGULARLY ALL OVER, again concentrating on the breasts, buttocks, belly, hips and thighs. This will keep skin healthy and supple, and encourage new skin growth and good circulation.

RECOMMENDED RECIPES: Avocado and Cumin Dip (page 180); Nut Butter (especially made with almonds, page 181); Fennel and Flaxseed Oatcakes (page 175).

Swelling

Many women notice swelling around their fingers, feet and ankles during the second and especially the third trimester. This is due to bodily fluid increasing until baby is born. If you are worried about drastic swelling, see your midwife, especially in later pregnancy, as this can be a symptom of pre-eclampsia. To help relieve this uncomfortable complaint:

KEEP UP YOUR FLUID INTAKE to flush excess fluids through your system.

AVOID ADDING SALT TO YOUR FOOD, as excess salt can contribute towards fluid retention.

ELEVATE YOUR FEET AND ANKLES WHEN SITTING to help drain fluid away from these areas.

REMOVE YOUR RINGS IF YOUR FINGERS SWELL to avoid discomfort.

EAT LEAFY GREEN VEGETABLES to avoid a developing a magnesium deficiency, which can result in oedema (fluid retention).

RECOMMENDED RECIPES: Green Minestrone (page 162); Rehydrater juice (page 208).

Balancing hormones

In order for our bodies to be working optimally, the two main female sex hormones, oestrogen and progesterone, need to be balanced and working in harmony. This is especially important while trying to conceive a baby and during pregnancy, when they will fluctuate. The '5 R's below are a way of ensuring our hormones are balanced, helping to boost fertility levels and make sure you're firing on all cylinders!

REMOVE sugary foods, additives, processed foods, caffeine and alcohol from your diet, which all have a negative impact on our gut and the good/bad bacteria within it, which in turn can affect our hormone levels if not functioning properly. These 'bad foods' also affect the liver and one of the processes it uses to detoxify oestrogens.

REPLACE LESS-NOURISHING FOOD WITH NOURISHING FOOD: remove processed foods from your diet and replace them with foods which will boost your oestrogen levels, such as brassicas and dark leafy vegetables. Aim for at least two servings per day. Try the Oestrogen Boost juice (page 208) first thing in the morning or as a mid-afternoon pick-me-up. Increase your protein intake in the form of eggs, lean white meat, fish, pulses, seeds and nuts, and up your vitamin C levels with healthy snacks of strawberries, kiwi fruit and fresh oranges, or have a Green Omega smoothie (page 209).

RE-INOCULATE: having replaced the bad with the good, continue to nourish the gut and ensure it receives all the right things. Add extra vitamin B6 in the form of dark leafy vegetables, and essential amino acids, which are necessary for hormone growth and found in oily fish. Try to eat oily fish twice a week and keep taking your omega-3 supplements – see the recipe for Miso Salmon with Edamame, Seaweed and Cucumber Salad on page 55.

REPAIR: in order for the liver to detoxify we need to make sure it is functioning at full capacity. Keep up your vitamin C intake and ensure your gut is healthy, as regular bowel movements are vital for expelling old oestrogen. Lots of filtered water and fibre in your diet will help with this – try the Rehydrator juice on page 208 and my Coconut and Banana Muffins on page 119.

REBALANCE: magnesium, otherwise known as nature's tranquilliser, is an essential mineral for supporting the adrenal gland, which controls the stress hormone cortisol. Magnesium promotes good sleep, relaxation and calm, and can be found in wholegrains, darky leafy vegetables, seeds and nuts – see my recipe for Sweet and Salty Munchy Seeds and Nuts on page 176, and try Super Seed Soda Bread (page 46) instead of your usual shop-bought bread. Vitamin B will also help support the adrenal gland and can be found in eggs, fish, lean white meats and many fresh vegetables.

Food hygiene

While pregnant, you are more vulnerable to the dangers of food poisoning. This might mean you fall ill due to a food-borne disease, which could potentially harm you and your baby; in very rare cases food poisoning can lead to serious complications, especially in the early stages of pregnancy. For this reason, it is important to be aware of food hygiene both in the home and when you are out. The following guidelines are those recommended by the UK Food Standards Agency and the NHS to promote good food hygiene and keep us all safe.

Wash your hands

Wash your hands thoroughly with soap and hot water, and dry them on a clean, dry cloth or some kitchen roll before handling food.

Be sure to wash your hands after handling raw foods, including meat, fish, eggs and vegetables, as well as after touching the bin, going to the toilet, blowing your nose or touching animals, including pets.

Keep your fridge below 5°C (40°F)

Keep your fridge temperature below 5°C (40°F). By keeping food cold you slow down the growth of illness-causing bacteria.

Keep raw meat separate

It's especially important to keep raw meat away from ready-to-eat foods such as salad, fruit and bread. This is because these foods won't be cooked before you eat them, so any bacteria that get on to them won't be killed. Always cover raw meat and store it on the bottom shelf of the fridge, where it can't touch other food or drip any juices on to it.

Defrost food properly

Ensure you fully defrost all food, including all pre-cooked meals, meat, fish and shellfish, in the bottom of your fridge overnight. Do not defrost in warm water in the sink, as this will encourage bacteria to grow and could make you sick. Never refreeze food that has already been defrosted.

Respect 'use-by' dates

Don't eat food that is past its 'use-by' date. These are based on scientific tests that show how quickly harmful bugs can develop in the packaged food.

Wash worktops

Wash worktops before and after preparing food, particularly when they've been touched by raw meat — including poultry — raw eggs, fish and vegetables. You can use an antibacterial spray or wipes, or hot soapy water.

Wash dishcloths

Wash dishcloths and tea towels regularly and let them dry before you use them again. Dirty, damp cloths are the perfect place for bacteria to breed. Use disposable kitchen roll when wiping down work surfaces as this can be thrown away after every use, reducing the risk of spreading bacteria.

Use separate chopping boards

Use separate chopping boards for raw food and ready-to-eat food. Raw foods can contain harmful bacteria that spread very easily to anything they touch, including other foods, worktops, chopping boards and knives. I have a red board for raw meat, a green one for raw vegetables and a general wooden board for all other foods, all of which I wash after each use in hot, soapy water.

Cook food thoroughly

Cook food thoroughly and check that it's piping hot all the way through. Make sure all meat, including red meat, poultry, pork, burgers, sausages and kebabs are cooked until steaming hot, with no pink meat inside.

Cool leftovers quickly

If you have cooked food that you're not going to eat straight away, cool it as quickly as possible (within 90 minutes) and store it in the fridge or freezer. Use any leftovers from the fridge within two days. You can cool food quickly by spreading it out in a large shallow tray or bowl to increase the surface area.

You can also cool pasta, eggs and fresh vegetables in ice-cold water.

Reheating food

If reheating food, ensure you heat it to at least 80°C (175°F) to destroy any bacteria present. Cooked rice, if left at room temperature for too long, will grow bacteria called Bacillus cereus, which can cause food poisoning and will not be destroyed by reheating. Try to eat rice as soon as it has been cooked, and if this isn't possible, cool it quickly and cover with cling film. Leave it in the fridge for no longer than two days. You can reheat rice if you have cooked it yourself, but never reheat rice from a take-away as you have no way of knowing if it has been reheated already: rice should never be reheated more than once. To reheat your own rice, place it in a glass bowl, cover with cling film and microwave until piping hot.

Sterilising jars for chutneys, jams and compotes

A few of the recipes in this book can be kept and stored in sterilised jars. It's important to sterilise jars properly, however, to avoid bacterial growth and contamination. To do this, heat the oven to 140°C (285°F). Wash the jars in hot, soapy water and rinse well. Place the jars on a baking tray and put them into the hot oven to dry off completely. If using Kilner jars, boil the rubber seal in water on the stove for 5 minutes as the heat from the oven may damage the seal.

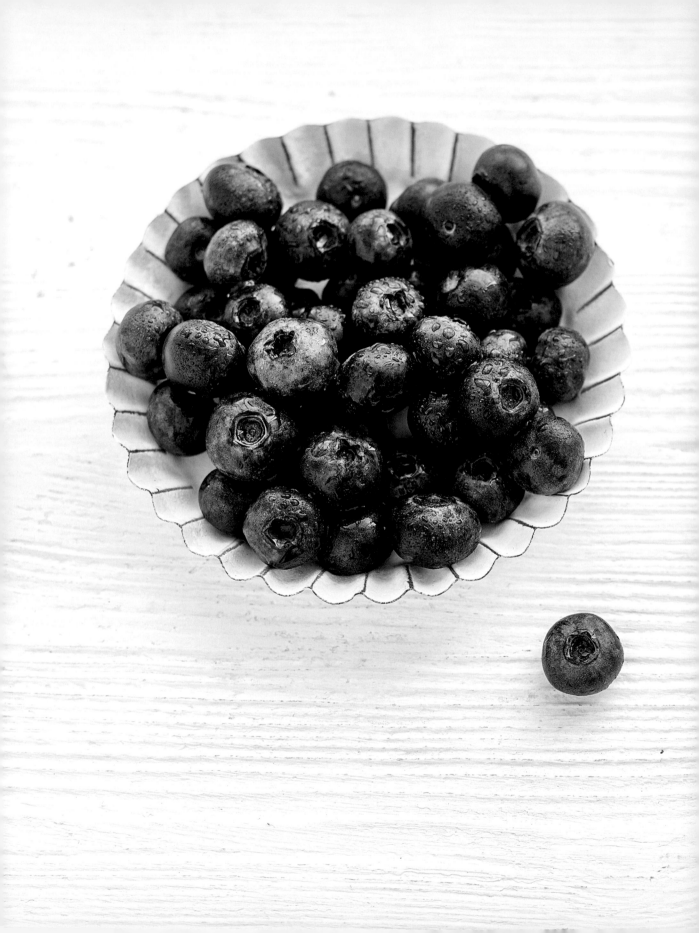

PRECONCEPTION

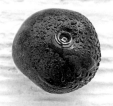

Food is so easily accessible these days that it's sometimes easy to overlook the fact that we aren't actually nourishing our bodies properly. A balanced and healthy diet is always essential; not drinking too much and cooking from scratch whenever you can. But while these are the obvious ways to get in good shape, there are many things we can eat to give ourselves the best possible chance of getting pregnant.

Eating well and being a healthy weight primes your body for baby-making, and a good diet will help you lay down the nutrient stores needed throughout your pregnancy when it does eventually happen. Pregnancy can put a huge strain on our bodies physically. Having a good and well-balanced diet can reduce our risk of getting sick, strengthen our immune systems and make us feel generally better, helping our bodies to function at full power.

If you have only recently started trying for a baby, please don't worry if it hasn't yet happened. NHS guidelines suggest that 84 per cent of couples will fall pregnant within their first year of having regular unprotected sex. Anything within this time frame is considered normal. For every 100 couples trying to conceive, 84 will succeed within the first year, 92 within two years, and 93 within three years. Don't forget that your lifestyle, age and weight will all affect your chances of conceiving.

I want to stress that trying to conceive can take time and there is no quick fix. But what the recipes in this chapter can do is help you to adopt a lifestyle that can boost your chances of falling pregnant. The recipes that follow combine all the necessary ingredients and food groups to help promote a healthier you. Taking the advice of nutritional therapist Henrietta Norton, I have developed recipes which are not only easy to create at home for the whole family, but also will ensure you are nourishing your body correctly, which will help support a healthy pregnancy.

I followed and cooked this collection of recipes while thinking about and trying for our baby. I truly believe that eating well, knowing exactly what I was putting into my body and why it was helping me, put me in a positive state of mind and health which helped me fall pregnant. I also felt great while cooking and eating these recipes – refreshed, healthy and energised.

What Does My Body Need And Why?

When trying for a baby it is important that your body is functioning at its full potential and that you are as fit and healthy as you can be in order to sustain the nine months of pregnancy. As well as being relaxed and in a good place mentally, it's really important that your diet and lifestyle are as clean and nutritionally rich as possible.

What to avoid

ALCOHOL: try to avoid drinking alcohol as much as possible. By all means have a drink with your dinner on special occasions, but be aware that drinking heavily and regularly will impact on your health and therefore might affect your ability to conceive.

SMOKING: smoking has been proven to reduce your chances of falling pregnant. A study published in the *Journal of Biosocial Science*, conducted by the Imperial Cancer Research Fund's general practice research group, showed clear links between smoking and fertility problems. The study suggested that the chances of conceiving are far higher among non-smokers than among those who smoke. However, it also suggested that it is never too late to give up, and that the chances of a former smoker conceiving are equal to those of a non-smoker after just one year.

Smoking has been shown to increase the risk of babies being small for their gestational age and the development of congenital heart defects in newborns (i). If you are trying for a baby, you should try to quit or at least cut back. This will also help when you do fall pregnant and need to stop smoking altogether.

CAFFEINE: caffeine reduces your body's ability to absorb nutrients and has been proven as a factor in low birth weight, which can lead to complications after birth (ii). It has also been proven to contribute towards miscarriage. Caffeine is present not only in tea and coffee but also in energy drinks, chocolate and certain types of flu medicine and other over-the-counter painkillers.

Try to limit your intake to 1–2 cups of tea or coffee per day, or even better, switch to decaffeinated.

Once you do fall pregnant, it is advised by the NHS that you limit yourself to 200mg of caffeine per day. This is the equivalent to two cups of instant coffee or medium-strength black tea.

A 2008 study published by Dr De-Kun Li in the *American Journal of Obstetrics and Gynecology* suggested that women who consumed more than 330mg of caffeine a day were twice as likely to miscarry than those who drank less than this amount.

i; ii: See page 224 for supporting information

What to include

FOLATE: proven to prevent spina bifida and reduce homocysteine, which is an amino acid. Recent research has shown that high levels of homocysteine have been associated with miscarriage (iii). The NHS advises that all women trying to conceive take 400mcg of folic acid per day and continue into week 12 of pregnancy. Folate is found in leafy green vegetables, pulses, wholegrains, seeds and nuts, so make sure you eat lots of these as well as taking your 400mcg supplement.

VITAMIN E: this antioxidant and anticoagulant has been shown to reduce the risk of miscarriage (iv). It is also said to support libido and fertility (v). Vitamin E is found in oily fish, seeds, avocados and peanuts.

MAGNESIUM: lack of magnesium (and potassium) in the diet has been shown to reduce fertility levels and increase possible risk of miscarriage (vi). To increase these minerals in your diet, eat wholegrains, pulses, dried fruits and nuts. Also, consider taking a good supplement (vi).

VITAMIN C: this has been shown to reduce the risk of DNA damage in the sperm and ovum (vii). Vitamin C is found in fresh tomatoes, oranges, peppers, strawberries, kiwi fruit and green vegetables, but it is easily destroyed through cooking so these foods are best eaten raw.

SELENIUM: an antioxidant that can prevent DNA damage and chromosome breakdown, which is a known cause of miscarriage and birth defects (viii). Ensure to eat oily fish, shellfish, avocados, wholegrains, seeds and nuts.

ZINC: controls hormone levels, which stimulate the ovaries and testes, and promotes the growth of the foetus. Zinc is found in pumpkin seeds, white fish, egg yolks, and wholemeal and rye bread.

OMEGA-3: many women don't eat enough oily fish and are therefore deficient in DHA and essential fatty acids. These fatty acids are needed for cell production in the ovaries. Eat plenty of oily fish (but no more than 2 portions per week), flaxseed oil, wholegrains, leafy green vegetables and nuts.

VITAMIN B12: this is needed for the uptake of folate and is essential for a healthy pregnancy. It is found in oily fish, cottage cheese, lean white meat and wholegrains such as brown rice.

VITAMIN B FAMILY (1, 2, 3, 5 AND 6): needed for equilibrium in the sex hormones, oestrogen and progesterone, and in sufficient amounts to build a healthy pregnancy. These hormone levels can be disrupted by lifestyle strains such as stress and anxiety, antibiotics and the contraceptive pill. Keep up your intake of wholegrains such as rye and quinoa, as well as fruits and vegetable, eggs and poultry.

iii; iv; v; vi; vii; viii: **See page 224 for supporting information**

IRON: low iron levels can affect fertility, and good levels of iron have been shown to protect against miscarriage and protect against low birth weight. Eat a balanced diet including leafy green vegetables, red meat, dried fruits and nuts.

BETA-CAROTENE: this is converted to vitamin A in the body and is needed for producing sex hormones, as well as helping to support normal functioning of the immune system and iron metabolism in mum, helping to support the developing embryo. Beta-carotene can be found in bright and colourful fruits and vegetables such as carrots, sweet potatoes, tomatoes, oranges, pumpkins and leafy green vegetables.

Trying to get pregnant can be a stressful time for couples and it can sometimes feel a bit like it is taking over your life. The key is to stay relaxed and allow nature to takes its course. Stay well rested, hydrated, exercise little and often, and eat a healthy diet and, most importantly, have lots of sex!

AVOCADO, BLUEBERRY AND FETA ON RYE

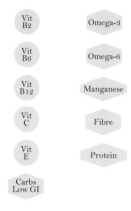

Vit B2 · Omega-3
Vit B6 · Omega-6
Vit B12 · Manganese
Vit C · Fibre
Vit E · Protein
Carbs Low GI

Avocados are something we should all have in our fruit bowl. Extremely rich in good fats, they provide excellent brain food and body fuel. In particular they are rich in omega-3 fatty acids, which help regulate your reproductive sex hormones, oestrogen and progesterone. It takes exactly nine months for an avocado to grow from blossom to ripened fruit ready for picking – if that's not nature's way of showing you a food that is good for fertility, I don't know what is!

Blueberries are one of nature's little superfoods, containing lots of magnesium, which helps regulate ovulation. Their natural tartness works really well with the richness of avocado and the saltiness of feta. You'll be surprised by how delicious and refreshing this breakfast is.

PREP TIME 10 MINUTES • SERVES 2

1 ripe avocado
100g pasteurised feta cheese
200g blueberries
zest and juice of 1 lime
½ green chilli, finely chopped
3 tbsp avocado oil or good quality extra virgin olive oil, plus extra to serve
4 slices rye bread or Super Seed Soda Bread (page 46)
10 fresh basil leaves
1 tbsp sunflower seeds
salt and freshly ground black pepper

1 Cut the avocado in half and remove the stone. Scoop out the flesh using a spoon and place it in a bowl. Mash gently with the back of a fork before crumbling in the feta, followed by the blueberries, lime zest and juice, chilli and avocado oil. Season with salt and pepper, stir to combine and leave to marinate while you toast your bread.

2 Tear the basil leaves into the avocado and blueberry mixture, then pile it on top of the warm toast and sprinkle with sunflower seeds. Drizzle with a little more avocado oil before serving.

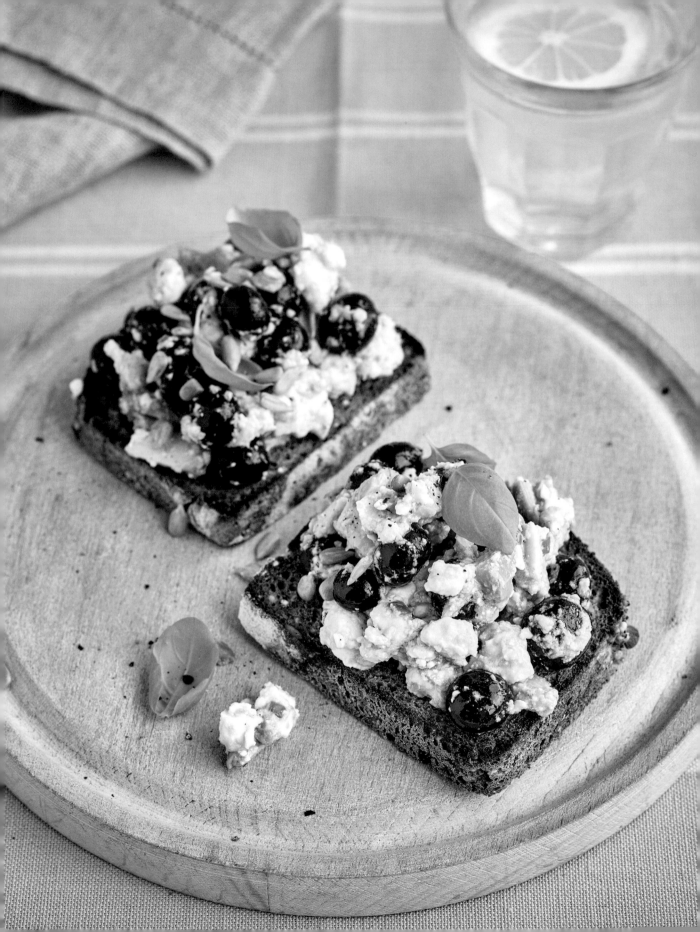

SUPER SEED SODA BREAD

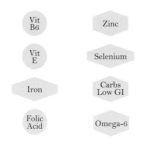

Vit B6

Vit E

Iron

Folic Acid

Zinc

Selenium

Carbs Low GI

Omega-6

This delicious bread contains no active yeast, and is much quicker to make than a standard bread recipe. I make a loaf and freeze it in slices, ready to be toasted and topped with all my favourite things. Currently this is Marmite and sliced tomato, but I'm sure that will change by next week! Cheese and honey is also a really great combination.

By making your own loaf, you can add all the essential ingredients your body needs in preparation for carrying a little one for a full nine months. Seeds and wholemeal flour have amazing qualities, such as helping to balance reproductive hormones. I bet you never thought you'd get that from a slice of bread!

PREP TIME 15 MINUTES • COOK TIME 1 HOUR, PLUS COOLING TIME
• MAKES 1 x 750G LOAF (12 SLICES)

250g spelt flour, or buckwheat or brown rice flour for gluten-free
250g wholemeal flour or gluten-free bread flour
2 tbsp baking powder
1 tsp salt
2 tbsp sunflower seeds
2 tbsp pumpkin seeds
2 tbsp sesame seeds
2 tbsp ground flaxseed
1 tbsp poppy seeds
100ml cows' milk, plus a little extra to brush on top of the loaf before baking
300ml buttermilk or natural yogurt

TO DECORATE
salt
extra seeds

1 Preheat the oven to 200°C (fan 180°C). Grease the inside of a 750g loaf tin with a little oil and coat lightly with flour.

2 Mix all the dry ingredients in a large bowl and make a well in the centre. Pour in the milk and buttermilk and bring everything together to form a dough. Work the dough by kneading it until all the ingredients are combined and the dough is smooth. It's really important not to overwork it, though, so as soon as it starts to stick together it's ready. Now form the dough into a loaf shape and place it in the loaf tin.

3 Use a sharp knife to make a long slit across the top of the loaf – this will help the dough to rise. Brush the top of the dough with a little milk and sprinkle with the extra seeds and a little salt. Bake in the oven for 1 hour. If the loaf is colouring too quickly simply cover it loosely with some foil.

4 Check to see if the bread is cooked by removing it from the tin and tapping its bottom. If it sounds hollow and doesn't look wet in any way, it is ready. If not, place the loaf back in the oven, out of its tin, for another 10 minutes or so. Leave to cool completely before slicing and eating or freezing. I prefer to eat mine toasted.

CHIA SEED AND OAT BREAKFAST POTS WITH STEWED APPLE COMPOTE

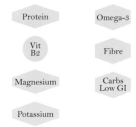

Protein

Vit B2

Magnesium

Potassium

Omega-3

Fibre

Carbs Low GI

Chia seeds have amazing nutritional qualities and are really easy to incorporate into your diet. Both white and black varieties are rich in omega-3, which is essential for cell production in the ovaries and maintaining a good balance of oestrogen and progesterone, and has been shown to reduce the risk of miscarriage. Omega-3 is also essential for healthy sperm, so get your partner to try this one as well.

This breakfast is best made the night before, to allow the chia seeds and oats to soak up all the milk. In the morning all you need to do is assemble it into a satisfying breakfast.

PREP TIME 5 MINUTES, PLUS OVERNIGHT SOAKING • SERVES 2

100g pinhead or rolled porridge oats
4 tbsp chia seeds
150ml milk of your choosing
zest of 1 orange
½ tsp ground cinnamon
2–3 tbsp runny honey

FOR THE APPLE COMPOTE
1 cooking apple, peeled and finely chopped
juice of ½ lemon
1 tbsp runny honey or agave nectar
pinch of ground cinnamon

TO SERVE
handful of blueberries or pumpkin seeds
runny honey

1 Start by making the compote. Place the chopped apple in a saucepan with the lemon juice, honey and cinnamon. Simmer over a low heat until the apple starts to break down – this will take about 5 minutes – stirring occasionally and adding a little water if it starts to look dry. Set aside to cool, then transfer to a lidded container and store in the fridge until you're ready to use it.

2 In a separate bowl, mix the oats with the chia seeds, milk, the orange zest, cinnamon and honey, cover with cling film and leave to soak overnight in the fridge.

3 When ready to serve the next morning, layer the soaked oat and chia seed mixture with the apple compote, then add a final drizzle of honey and half a handful of pumpkin seeds or blueberries to each bowl.

QUINOA PORRIDGE WITH BANANA, PEAR AND CINNAMON

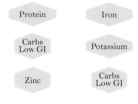

Protein

Iron

Carbs Low GI

Potassium

Zinc

Carbs Low GI

Quinoa has become a real staple of mine, and not just while just trying for our baby. It's a really versatile ingredient and one that can be used in lots of different savoury and sweet recipes. It's also a great source of protein, so essential for helping keep you strong and healthy. I always make my porridge with almond milk, as I think it adds a delicious creaminess and nutty flavour. Almond milk is very high in B vitamins and iron, which can help guard your body against miscarriage.

COOK TIME 25 MINUTES • SERVES 2

80g quinoa
200ml almond milk
  or cows' milk
150ml water
1 tsp ground cinnamon
2 tbsp runny honey
1 pear, skin on and grated
1 banana, mashed

TO SERVE
1 tbsp pumpkin seeds
2 tsp milled flaxseed or
  sesame seeds

1 Wash the quinoa under cold water and place in a saucepan. Pour over the milk and water and add the cinnamon, then bring to the boil over a medium heat. Once boiling, reduce the heat and leave to gently simmer for 15–20 minutes, stirring regularly to stop it sticking to the bottom of the pan. Add the honey and stir well.

2 Add in the grated pear and mashed banana, stirring them through before dividing the porridge between bowls. Top with the seeds and serve.

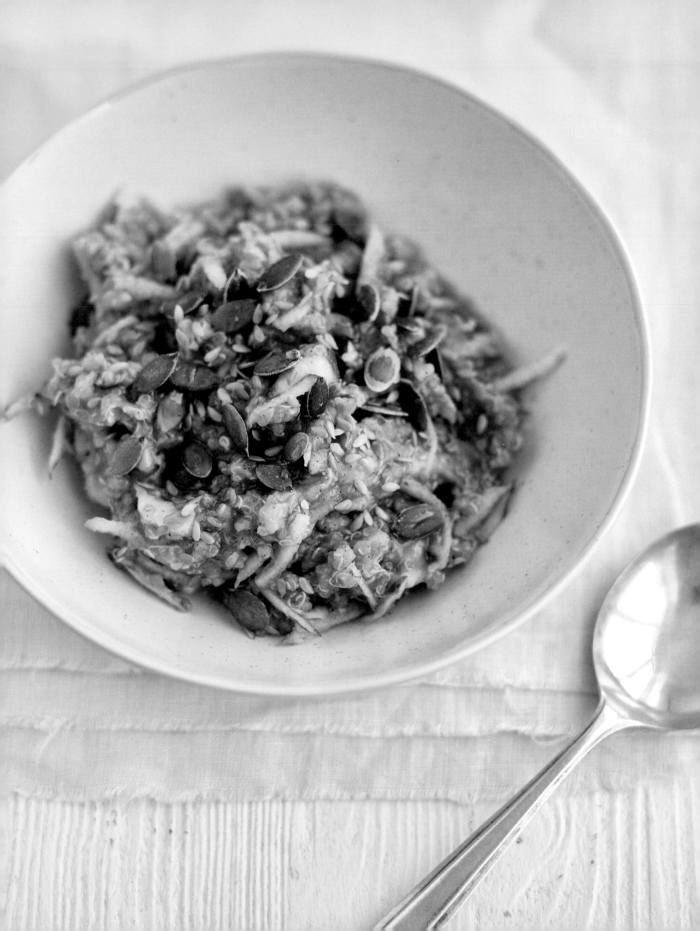

QUICK BOSTON BEANS ON SEEDY TOAST

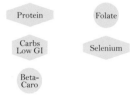

Protein

Folate

Carbs
Low GI

Selenium

Beta-
Caro

This isn't a traditional Boston Beans recipe. I've shortened it significantly and tried to put a slightly healthier twist on it, using molasses instead of the traditional treacle, as molasses is extremely high in B vitamins. It is available in most supermarkets and can be used in place of treacle in all recipes. Beans are fabulous ingredients to use in cooking, especially when making breakfast or brunch. They are a brilliant source of protein so keep you going until lunchtime, as well as being high in folate.

PREP TIME 5 MINUTES (PLUS OVERNIGHT SOAKING IF USING DRIED BEANS) •
COOK TIME 20 MINUTES TO 3 HOURS, DEPENDING ON YOUR METHOD • SERVES 4

450g dried haricot beans,
 or 2 x 400g tins
 cooked beans
1 tsp English mustard
 powder
1 tbsp molasses
1 tbsp dark brown sugar
1 tbsp tomato purée
small pinch of ground cloves
125g smoked streaky bacon
1 tbsp Worcestershire sauce
500ml chicken stock
salt and freshly ground
 black pepper

TO SERVE
4 tbsp stale breadcrumbs
4 tbsp grated
 Parmesan cheese
2 tbsp rapeseed oil
4 thick slices seedy bread,
 or make your own
 Super Seed Soda
 Bread (page 46)

1 If using dried beans, leave them to soak overnight in plenty of cold water.

2 Mix the mustard powder, molasses, brown sugar, tomato purée and ground cloves together to form a paste.

3 Heat a large casserole pan over a medium heat and add the bacon. Cook for 4–5 minutes, until the fat starts to render out of the meat and the bacon is golden. Add the mustard paste and mix well. Now drain the beans, add them to the dish and stir to combine.

4 Pour over the Worcestershire sauce and stock, and bring to the boil. Simmer the beans until they are soft and have absorbed some of the liquid. If you are using dried beans, this will take up to 1 hour; if using tinned, it will be as little as 20 minutes. You can also cook the beans in the oven at 170°C (fan 150°C) for up to 3 hours – this will make for a really rich sauce if you have the time. Season with salt and pepper.

5 While your beans are cooking, preheat the oven to 200°C (fan 180°C) – if you are cooking your beans in the oven, save this step until the beans are cooked. Mix the breadcrumbs with the grated Parmesan in a bowl. Drizzle with the oil and scatter on to a baking tray. Bake in the oven for 8–10 minutes, until golden. Remove from the oven and set aside.

6 Once the beans are cooked, toast the bread. Spoon over the Boston Beans and sprinkle the Parmesan breadcrumbs over the top. Serve straight away.

PAN-ROASTED BEETROOT ON RYE

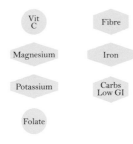

Vit C

Fibre

Magnesium

Iron

Potassium

Carbs Low GI

Folate

Beetroot, with its sweet earthy flavours, works really well with boiled eggs and this dish makes a really nutritious lunch or light supper. It is rich in vitamin C, folate, potassium and magnesium, helping your body lay down a good supply of these essential vitamins and minerals that it will need during your pregnancy. The leaves are the part of the vegetable that contain the most goodness, so try to buy beetroots with the green tops still on and stir these through pasta or steam them with your greens at dinner time.

PREP TIME 10 MINUTES • COOK TIME 20–30 MINUTES • SERVES 2

2 medium beetroots, skin on and trimmed (reserve the green tops)
4 free-range eggs
2 tbsp avocado oil, plus extra to serve
2 tbsp balsamic vinegar
2 tbsp finely chopped chives
4 slices rye bread or Super Seed Soda Bread (page 46)
4 anchovy fillets (optional)
salt and freshly ground black pepper

1 Start by preparing the beetroots. Place a large saucepan of cold water on the stove and season well with salt. Put the beetroots in the pan, skins on to prevent them from bleeding into the water, and bring to the boil. Cook for 20–30 minutes until tender.

2 While the beetroots are cooking, boil the eggs for 10 minutes in the same pan. Once cooked, remove from the pan and cool under the tap. Peel and roughly chop.

3 Once the beetroots are cooked, remove them from the water and leave to cool slightly. Wearing a pair of protective gloves (to prevent your hands getting stained), peel the beetroots using a small knife and dice them into 1cm pieces.

4 Pour the avocado oil and balsamic vinegar into a frying pan set over a medium heat. When hot, add the beetroot along with the beetroot tops, if you have them. Cook these for 3–4 minutes, until the beetroot has warmed through and slightly caramelised in the dressing and the tops are wilted.

5 Season with salt and pepper and add the chopped egg, along with the chopped chives. Mix well and coat in all the pan juices. Remove from the heat.

6 Toast the bread and drizzle with a little more avocado oil. Spoon on the egg and beetroot mixture and lay the anchovy fillets over the top (if you are having them).

HALLOUMI, LENTIL AND ROASTED PEPPER SALAD WITH RYE CROUTONS

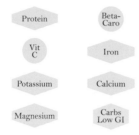

Protein

Beta-Caro

Vit C

Iron

Potassium

Calcium

Magnesium

Carbs Low GI

Halloumi will provide you with a good supply of calcium, as well as tasting delicious. Buy good quality halloumi and, if eating it while pregnant, make sure it has been pasteurised. The pepperiness of the watercress freshens up this whole dish. Watercress is a leaf I can't recommend enough – ditch the iceberg lettuce and switch to watercress as it's so rich in vitamin B6, which will help to support hormonal equilibrium, and magnesium, which can play a role in ovulation.

PREP TIME 15 MINUTES • COOK TIME 25 MINUTES • SERVES 2

100g uncooked Puy lentils, or 200g cooked/tinned lentils
3 tbsp rapeseed oil
2 garlic cloves, squashed but not peeled
2 slices stale rye or wholemeal or seeded bread
150g halloumi cheese, cut into 2cm pieces
12–15 baby plum tomatoes, halved
2 large roasted red peppers, sliced (homemade or from a jar)
2–3 large handfuls of washed baby watercress
salt and freshly ground black pepper

FOR THE DRESSING
2 tsp Dijon mustard
2 tbsp sherry vinegar
3 tbsp rapeseed oil
salt and freshly ground black pepper

1 If you need to cook your lentils, do this first. Wash them in cold water until the water runs clear. Transfer to a saucepan and cover with double the amount of water. Place the pan on the stove and bring to the boil before turning down the heat and simmering for 10–15 minutes until the lentils are tender. Once cooked, drain and season with a little salt. Put the cooked lentils into a bowl.

2 Now make your dressing. Combine all the ingredients in a small jar, season and place on the lid. Shake well for about 20 seconds until the dressing is combined and emulsified. Pour half over the warm lentils.

3 Heat a large frying pan and add 2 tablespoons of rapeseed oil. Add the squashed garlic and tear in the stale bread in bite-sized pieces, then toast in the oil for 5–6 minutes until golden brown. Remove the croutons from the pan and drain on a piece of kitchen roll.

4 Add the remaining oil and fry the halloumi until it turns slightly golden – this will take around 2 minutes per side. Now add the halved tomatoes and sliced peppers and heat through before stirring in the cooked lentils.

5 Place the watercress in a large serving bowl and pour over the hot halloumi, tomatoes, peppers and lentils. Season with pepper and pour over the remaining dressing. Top with the toasted croutons before tossing well and serving warm.

ROASTED CAULIFLOWER, QUINOA, ALMOND AND APRICOT SALAD

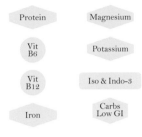

Protein

Vit B6

Vit B12

Iron

Magnesium

Potassium

Iso & Indo-3

Carbs Low GI

Cauliflower is such an under-used vegetable. We tend only to have it steamed or boiled or under a cheese sauce, but it has so much more potential! Rich in vitamin C, which helps to protect cells and keep them healthy, it increases the absorption of iron and reduces DNA damage in the ovum and sperm. Quinoa is the perfect vehicle for a salad like this, as it absorbs huge amounts of flavour with very little effort. It's a great source of protein and high in vitamin B12. People's B12 levels are often depleted by lifestyle factors such as fertility medication, the contraceptive pill and stress, so this is a great dish to get you back on track.

PREP TIME 15 MINUTES • COOK TIME 20 MINUTES • SERVES 2

FOR THE ROASTED CAULIFLOWER
1 tsp ground cumin
pinch of dried chilli flakes
1 tsp ground coriander
drizzle of rapeseed oil
½ cauliflower head, cut into small florets
salt and freshly ground black pepper

FOR THE SALAD
80g uncooked quinoa
30g flat-leaf parsley, finely chopped
2 tbsp flaked almonds, toasted
1 tbsp poppy seeds
100g dried apricots, chopped (look for the darker unsulphured ones)

FOR THE DRESSING
zest and juice of 2 lemons
1 tbsp apple cider vinegar
2 tsp Dijon mustard
3 tbsp good quality rapeseed oil
2 tsp runny honey

1 Preheat the oven to 200°C (fan 180°C). For the roasted cauliflower, place the spices and rapeseed oil in a large bowl, then add the cauliflower florets and toss everything together. Season with a little salt and pepper, and spread out on a baking sheet, then cook in the oven for 15 minutes.

2 While the cauliflower is roasting, cook the quinoa for the salad in boiling salted water for 10–12 minutes, until tender. Once cooked, drain and leave to one side.

3 Make the dressing by combining all the ingredients in a small jar, put the lid on and shake hard.

4 Pour the quinoa into a large mixing bowl and add the roasted cauliflower, along with the chopped parsley, toasted almonds, poppy seeds and chopped apricots. Mix well before adding the dressing to the warm salad. This salad is perfect served on its own, or with a piece of roasted salmon for an extra hit of omega-3.

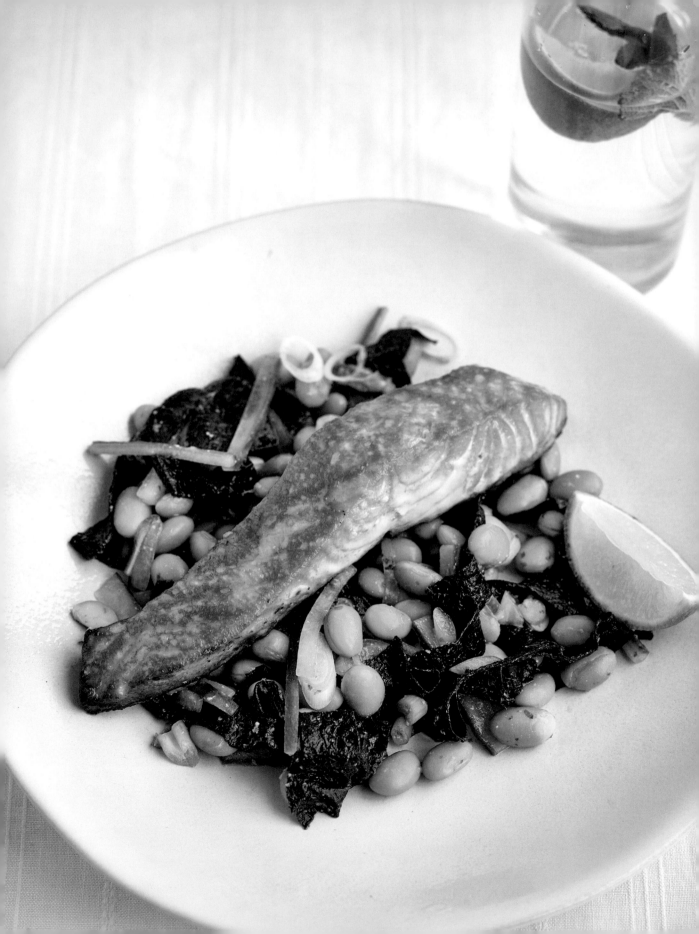

MISO SALMON WITH EDAMAME, SEAWEED AND CUCUMBER SALAD

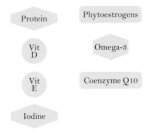

Protein
Phytoestrogens
Vit D
Omega-3
Vit E
Coenzyme Q10
Iodine

Just by reading the title of this dish, you know it is going to be good for you! Miso and seaweed are becoming more and more popular as cooking ingredients, and both are now easily obtainable. Keep them in the fridge or cupboard to add instant flavour to a whole host of dishes. Eight in ten women are thought to be deficient in omega-3, which is needed for cell production in the ovaries. Salmon is bursting with it and will count towards your recommended 1–2 portions of oily fish per week.

PREP TIME 20 MINUTES • COOK TIME 10 MINUTES • SERVES 4

2 tbsp white miso paste
2 tbsp reduced salt
    soy sauce
1 tbsp runny honey
4 salmon fillets, skin on
2 tbsp rapeseed oil

FOR THE SALAD
3 sheets nori (available
    in supermarkets)
3 handfuls of edamame
    or soya beans, podded
2 spring onions, trimmed
    and finely sliced
1 large cucumber, deseeded
    and cut into matchsticks

FOR THE DRESSING
1 tbsp white miso paste
1 tbsp mirin (Japanese
    sweet rice wine)
1 tbsp rice wine vinegar
2 tbsp runny honey
2cm piece fresh ginger,
    peeled and finely grated

TO SERVE
4 wedges of lime

1 Start by preparing the salmon. Mix the miso paste with the soy sauce and the honey, and rub all over the fish. Leave to marinate for a few minutes.

2 For the salad, soak the nori sheets in water for 1 minute, then cut them into strips about 2cm wide. Put the nori strips, edamame, spring onion and cucumber into a large bowl and stir to combine.

3 Whisk together the ingredients for the dressing in a bowl and pour over the salad.

4 Cook the fish by heating a frying pan over a high heat and adding the rapeseed oil. Lay the salmon in the hot oil and fry for 3–4 minutes per side, or until cooked through. Once they are cooked, remove from the heat and serve with the salad, pouring over the dressing from the bottom of the bowl, and a wedge of lime.

TRAY-BAKED COD WITH TOMATOES, CHICKPEAS AND KALE

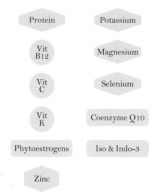

Protein

Potassium

Vit B12

Magnesium

Vit C

Selenium

Vit K

Coenzyme Q10

Phytoestrogens

Iso & Indo-3

Zinc

Chickpeas are a welcome substitute for potatoes in an evening meal. They contain many vital nutrients, including magnesium and potassium, deficiencies in which are associated with female infertility. Kale and courgettes are green, and therefore good for you! Kale is king when it comes to iron and iron plays a central role in the process of cell division involved in healthy fertility, as well as normal oxygen transport and a healthy immune system.

PREP TIME 15 MINUTES • COOK TIME 30 MINUTES • SERVES 4

2 x 400g tins chickpeas, rinsed and drained
400ml tomato juice or 300ml tomato passata mixed with 100ml water
¼ tsp smoked paprika
pinch of dried chilli flakes
200g baby plum tomatoes, halved
2 courgettes, cut into rough 3cm chunks
2–3 large handfuls of curly kale, roughly chopped
4 x 175g skinless cod fillets
2 tbsp rapeseed oil
30g Parmesan cheese, grated, plus extra to serve
salt and freshly ground black pepper

TO SERVE
30g flat-leaf parsley, finely chopped
4 handfuls of rocket or watercress leaves
1 lemon, cut into wedges

1 Preheat the oven to 200°C (fan 180°C). Take a large, high-sided, ovenproof dish and put in the chickpeas, tomato juice, paprika and dried chilli flakes. Mix together well and season with salt and pepper. Add the tomatoes and courgettes, along with the kale. Mix again to coat everything in the tomato juice.

2 Cook in the oven for 15 minutes, until the sauce starts to bubble and the kale begins to wilt. When this happens, give everything a good stir.

3 Rub the fish with the oil and a little salt and pepper. Lay the fish on top of the chickpea mixture and turn the oven up to 220°C (fan 200°C). Scatter the Parmesan over the top and bake for 15 minutes.

4 Once the fish is cooked – it should start to flake when pushed gently – remove the dish from the oven and scatter over the parsley and a little more grated Parmesan.

5 Serve with the salad leaves and lemon wedges.

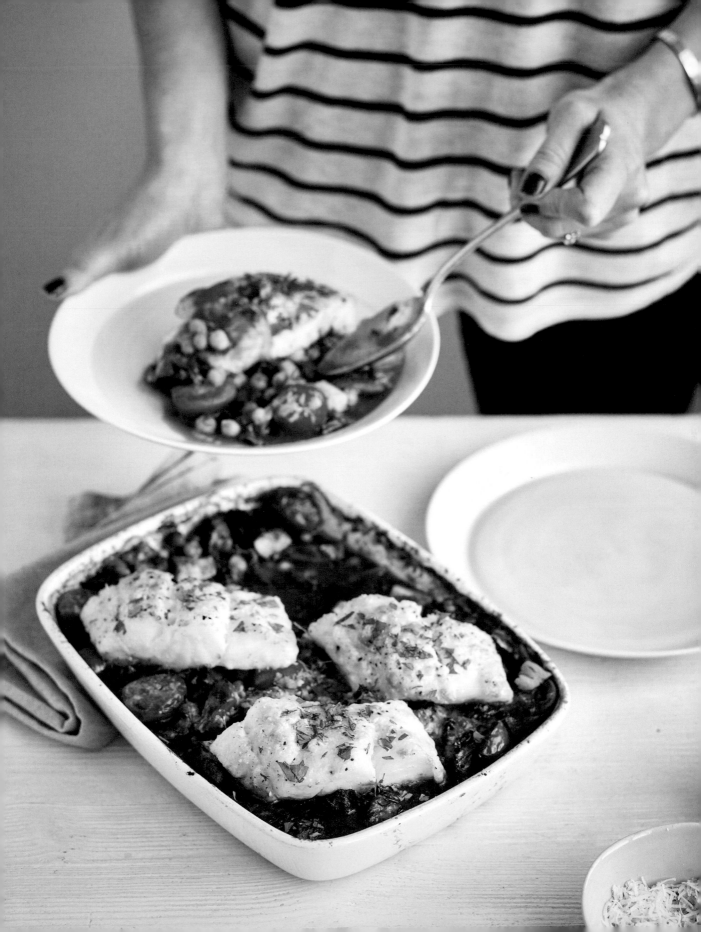

CHICKEN SATAY WITH PEANUTS AND CUCUMBER SALAD

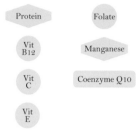

Protein

Vit B12

Vit C

Vit E

Folate

Manganese

Coenzyme Q10

A quick dish combining delicious moist chicken satay with moreish peanuts and refreshing cucumber. Peanuts are a great source of folate, which is needed for the healthy development of the baby's spinal cord and it is advised that all women who are trying to conceive take a daily supplement to build up their stores.

PREP TIME 25 MINUTES • COOK TIME 20–25 MINUTES • SERVES 2

6–8 free-range chicken mini fillets, or 2 chicken breasts cut into strips

FOR THE PEANUT SAUCE AND MARINADE
3 tbsp unsweetened crunchy peanut butter
2 tbsp agave nectar
1 tsp dried chilli flakes, or 1 fresh red chilli, finely chopped
200ml coconut milk
3 tbsp soy sauce
juice of 1 lime
5cm piece fresh ginger, peeled and grated
1 garlic clove, peeled and grated
salt and freshly ground black pepper

FOR THE CUCUMBER SALAD
1 large cucumber
1 large handful of bean sprouts
2 tbsp rice wine vinegar
2 tbsp plain peanuts, chopped and toasted
15g fresh mint or Thai basil leaves
salt

1 Soak 6–8 wooden skewers in water for a few minutes to prevent them from burning when you grill the chicken.

2 Combine all the ingredients for the sauce in a bowl, which will also be the marinade. Take one quarter of the sauce and place it in a separate large bowl along with the chicken. Mix well, cover and leave to marinate for 20 minutes.

3 Pour the remaining sauce into a small saucepan and bring to the boil. Allow to simmer for 10 minutes until thickened. Cover and set aside.

4 Make the salad by peeling the cucumber and cutting it in half lengthways. Use a spoon to scoop out the seeds and slice each half into crescent moons. Place in a bowl along with the bean sprouts, rice wine vinegar and peanuts. Season with a little salt.

5 Preheat the grill to medium.

6 Skewer each marinated chicken fillet on to a soaked wooden skewer, weaving the chicken so that it stays in place. Lay the chicken on a baking tray and cook under the preheated grill for 6–7 minutes on each side, until golden and cooked through.

7 Mix the mint or Thai basil into the cucumber salad, then serve alongside the chicken satay with the hot peanut sauce on the side.

TURKEY, SPINACH AND COURGETTE PATTIES WITH WILD RICE SALAD

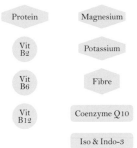

Protein

Vit B2

Vit B6

Vit B12

Magnesium

Potassium

Fibre

Coenzyme Q10

Iso & Indo-3

This recipe is great for lunch or dinner. I often make double the quantity so that I know I have a delicious and nutritious meal in the fridge for the next day. Turkey is an ingredient that isn't so commonly used, but turkey mince is widely available in supermarkets. It's a great flavour carrier as well as a good source of protein and vitamin B12, which we need to maximise our uptake of folate. You could also also use pork mince, which is a good source of coenzyme Q10.

PREP TIME 25 MINUTES • COOK TIME 20 MINUTES • SERVES 4

600g turkey mince
2 courgettes, grated
2 handfuls of baby leaf
    spinach, roughly chopped
zest of 1 lemon
1 tsp ground cumin
pinch of dried chilli flakes
1 free-range egg white
100g sesame seeds
4 tbsp rapeseed oil
salt and freshly ground
    black pepper

FOR THE RICE SALAD
100g wild or red rice
100g cracked bulgur wheat
50g flaked almonds
2 tbsp poppy seeds or
    sesame seeds
2 tbsp pumpkin seeds
zest and juice of 2 lemons
3 tbsp walnut or hazelnut oil
2 tbsp sultanas (golden
    raisins are also lovely)
30g flat-leaf parsley,
    roughly chopped
30g fresh mint leaves,
    roughly chopped
2 tsp sumac (optional)

TO SERVE
natural yogurt
4 lemon wedges

1 First make the salad by boiling the wild rice and the cracked wheat until tender but still with a slight bite. I usually do this in separate pans, as the wild rice takes longer (about 20 minutes) than the cracked wheat (about 10–12 minutes). Once cooked, drain the grains and place both into a large mixing bowl. Add in all the remaining salad ingredients, mix well and set aside.

2 Now place the turkey mince in a separate mixing bowl, along with the courgette, spinach, lemon zest, cumin and chilli flakes. Mix well, season with salt and pepper, and mould the mixture into 12 small patties. Coat each one with a little egg white, then roll in or sprinkle generously with the sesame seeds so they are coated all over.

3 Gently heat the rapeseed oil in a frying pan and add the patties in 2 batches (or more if needed), so as not to overcrowd the pan. Cook them until well coloured on each side, but keep the heat low so that they cook slowly, all the way through to the middle. They will need around 5 minutes per side. Place them onto a warmed plate and cover with foil while you cook the next batch.

4 Serve the hot patties with the rice salad, a good dollop of natural yogurt and a wedge of lemon on the side.

SMOKED HADDOCK 'RISOTTO' WITH A SOFT-BOILED EGG

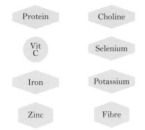

Protein

Vit C

Iron

Zinc

Choline

Selenium

Potassium

Fibre

Risotto is one of my favourite things. It's so comforting, and is extra tasty if you make it with a grain rather than with rice – especially pearl barley and spelt, which have delicious nutty flavours and really great textures.

Meanwhile, haddock and egg yolk contain high levels of zinc, which will help contribute towards a healthy body and therefore a better chance of conceiving.

PREP TIME 15 MINUTES, PLUS 20 MINUTES TO SOAK THE BARLEY AND SPELT
• COOK TIME 40–50 MINUTES • SERVES 4

250g pearl barley
100g spelt
400ml semi-skimmed
  cows' milk
600g skinless undyed
  smoked haddock fillets
1.5 litres chicken or
  vegetable stock
2 tbsp rapeseed oil
2 shallots, peeled and
  finely chopped
2 celery sticks, finely
  chopped
2 large leeks, trimmed
  and sliced
2 garlic cloves, peeled
  and finely chopped
200ml white wine
200g kale, torn into pieces
4 free-range eggs
30g Parmesan cheese,
  grated, plus extra to serve
zest of 2 lemons
2 tbsp crème fraîche
salt and freshly ground
  black pepper

1 Place the pearl barley and spelt in a bowl, cover with cold water and leave to soak for 20 minutes. Drain and set aside.

2 Pour the milk into a large high-sided frying pan and add the haddock fillets (it doesn't matter if the fish isn't completely covered). Bring to the boil over a medium heat, then turn off the heat, cover and leave the fish to gently poach in the hot milk while you make the 'risotto'.

3 Bring the stock up to a simmer in a large saucepan, then turn off the heat and cover. Heat the rapeseed oil in a large sauté pan over a high heat, then add the shallots, celery and leeks. Reduce the heat to low and cook for 4–5 minutes, stirring occasionally. Add the garlic and barley and spelt. Stir and let the grains toast for a few minutes before turning up the heat to medium and adding the white wine.

4 Once almost all of the wine has been absorbed (3–4 minutes), add one quarter of the hot stock. Stir every so often until most of the liquid has been absorbed – about 10–12 minutes over a medium heat. Repeat this process in 3 more batches with the rest of the stock, adding the kale with the last of the stock.

5 While the 'risotto' is cooking, bring a saucepan of water to the boil, lower in the eggs with a spoon, then leave them to boil for 6 minutes. Drain and peel straight away.

6 When the 'risotto' is ready (it will retain a slight bite, as spelt and barley don't go as soft as rice), flake in the poached haddock. Gently stir in the grated Parmesan, lemon zest and the crème fraîche. Season with lots of black pepper and a little salt. Cut the eggs in half and serve on top.

HARISSA LAMB MEATBALLS WITH BULGUR WHEAT SALAD

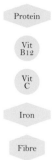

Protein

Vit B12

Vit C

Iron

Fibre

This dish pops up time and again in our house, always in a slightly different version depending on what I happen to have in the fridge. I find serving meatballs with bulgur wheat, rather than pasta, transforms an otherwise common and perhaps slightly predictable dish into something really exciting and different.

Bulgur wheat contains slow-releasing and nourishing carbohydrates, which will sustain you for longer, and magnesium, which plays a role in healthy cell division. It is also a good source of fibre and iron – one portion of this salad contains 10 per cent of your daily recommended dose. Lamb is a brilliant source of vitamin B12, which will maximise your folate uptake.

PREP TIME 20 MINUTES • COOK TIME 20 MINUTES • SERVES 2–3

400g minced lamb
2–3 tbsp harissa paste
2 tbsp rapeseed oil
12 cherry tomatoes, halved
salt and freshly ground
    black pepper

FOR THE SALAD
75g bulgur wheat
2 large vine tomatoes,
    deseeded and finely
    chopped
½ cucumber, deseeded
    and finely chopped
½ red onion, finely chopped
100g pasteurised feta
    cheese, crumbled
15g fresh mint leaves,
    finely chopped
15g fresh coriander
    leaves, finely chopped
zest and juice of 1 lemon
2 tsp sumac
2–3 tbsp extra virgin
    rapeseed oil or extra
    virgin olive oil
salt and freshly ground
    black pepper

TO SERVE
1 tsp harissa paste
3 tbsp natural yogurt
2–3 lemon wedges

1 Put the lamb mince into a bowl, add the harissa paste and season with salt and pepper. Mix everything together well, then mould the mixture into about 12–16 meatballs – I normally make them a little smaller than a golf ball. Place the meatballs on a plate, cover in cling film and put in the fridge while you prepare the bulgur wheat salad.

2 Boil the bulgur wheat in boiling salted water for 10 minutes until tender. Remove from the heat and drain well. Transfer to a large bowl.

3 Mix the tomatoes, cucumber, onion, feta, mint and coriander with the warm bulgur wheat, then stir in the lemon zest and juice, sumac and oil. Season with salt and pepper.

4 Place a large frying pan over a high heat and add the rapeseed oil. When it is hot, add in the meatballs and fry for 6–8 minutes until they start to turn golden; move them about a bit in the pan, but do so gently as they may start to break up. Add the cherry tomatoes to the pan and cook for another 6–8 minutes, until the tomatoes start to break down and form a loose sauce.

5 Before serving, mix the harissa paste with the yogurt. I like to just ripple the harissa in the top of the yogurt as it looks very pretty. Serve the bulgur wheat with the meatballs spooned over the top, and the yogurt and lemon wedges on the side.

VIETNAMESE BEEF SALAD WITH CITRUS DRESSING

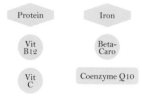

Protein Iron

Vit B12 Beta-Caro

Vit C Coenzyme Q10

This refreshing and vibrant salad is perfect for a quick, healthy and flavoursome lunch or dinner. Beef is iron-rich, and carrots not only contain beta-carotene – essential for a strong immune system – but are the perfect contrast for the rich beef and sharp dressing. Finish the salad by smothering it with crunchy sesame seeds, which contain coenzyme Q10, good levels of which can lead to increased likelihood of conception.

PREP TIME 20 MINUTES • COOK TIME 10 MINUTES • SERVES 2

300–400g lean beef steak
2 tbsp soy sauce
2 tbsp rapeseed oil

FOR THE SALAD
3 large carrots, peeled and cut into matchsticks (or you can use a spiralizer)
2 handfuls of bean sprouts
2 spring onions, trimmed and cut into matchsticks
10–12 fresh mint leaves
2 tbsp sesame seeds, toasted

FOR THE DRESSING
1 bird's eye chilli, finely chopped (leave the seeds in if you like it hot)
5cm piece fresh ginger, peeled and cut into matchsticks
1 tsp agave nectar or caster sugar
juice of 2 limes
2 tbsp reduced salt light soy sauce
2 tsp fish sauce

TO SERVE
1 tbsp sesame seeds
1 tsp sesame oil

1 Put a griddle pan over a very high heat. While it is heating up, sprinkle the steak with the soy sauce, then rub it all over with the oil. Lay the steak in the hot pan – it needs to be extremely hot to get nice chargrill lines across the steak – and cook to your liking; as a guide, a 1.5–2cm-thick steak will need around 4–5 minutes on each side to cook it medium rare. Transfer the steak to a warm plate and leave uncovered to rest while you make the salad.

2 Combine the carrots in a bowl with the bean sprouts, spring onions and mint leaves. Mix well.

3 Make the dressing by whisking all the ingredients together in a bowl. Taste to check you are happy with the flavours. You may need a little more soy or sweetness, depending on your preferences – the dressing should be a good balance of salt, sweet, sour and spice. Pour the dressing over the carrot salad before adding the sesame seeds.

4 To serve, slice the steak into thin strips and place them on top of the salad. Sprinkle over a few more sesame seeds and drizzle over a little sesame oil to finish.

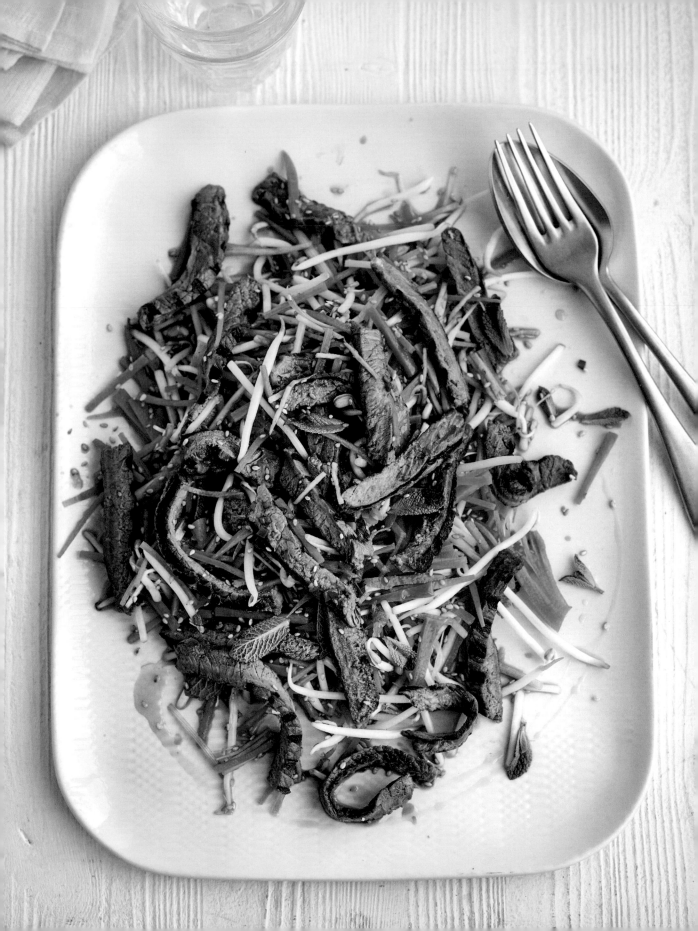

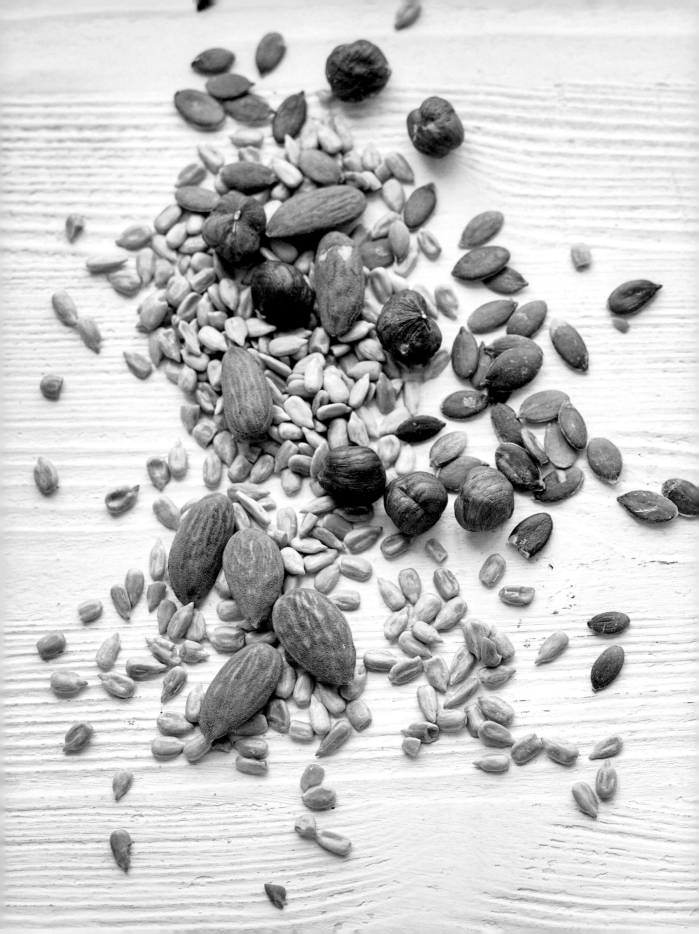

FIRST TRIMESTER

Congratulations! This may be the second recipes chapter, but I can assure you that it's the first chapter of the rest of your life. Once you see that little line appear on the pregnancy test, your whole life instantly changes! With no longer just yourself to look after, healthy eating will become something that I'm sure you will be very keen to embrace. Choosing to eat a well-balanced and healthy diet while pregnant will have a positive effect on you and your baby for the rest of your lives.

Your body will be working extra hard to absorb all the relevant nutrients from your normal daily food, to ensure the little one inside you is growing as he or she should. Without a healthy and well-balanced diet, your body will be forced to work even harder, leaving you even more exhausted.

Despite what many people often say, you are not eating for two. In fact, you need no extra calories until you are six months pregnant and in the third trimester of pregnancy, when you need only an extra 200 calories per day – the equivalent of a slice of toast and a banana.

In the first trimester, it can feel a bit like you have the worst hangover you have ever experienced. At least that's how I felt. Extreme tiredness and sickness can hit you in great waves when you are least expecting it. This is caused by changing hormones, but once the placenta has developed and taken over the job your hormones are doing, you should start to feel better (usually around weeks 12–16).

Morning sickness differs from woman to woman and doesn't just occur in the morning, despite its name. For some, it can continue throughout the entire pregnancy and no one is really sure why. In very unfortunate cases, women can suffer with a condition called hyperemesis gravidarum. This causes excessive vomiting and nausea throughout pregnancy and can lead to hospitalisation to replenish fluids lost through sickness. This type of sickness usually presents itself at around weeks 4–5 and lasts longer than the usual 6–8 weeks.

So what's this chapter all about, if most of the time you feel like putting your head down a toilet or crawling under the duvet until it's all over? Well, women can feel anxious about not wanting to eat certain foods during the first 12 weeks of pregnancy. This chapter will show you that, at this stage, a little can go a long way, and you don't need to force yourself to eat copious amounts of kale if you don't feel like it. Also included in this chapter are recipes to help reduce the symptoms of morning sickness or at least keep them at bay for a while, and recipes to provide nourishment for you and baby without you having to spend hours in the kitchen cooking and clearing up.

During my first trimester I only wanted carbohydrates, and many women find they feel utterly ravenous all the time. It's important to keep your blood sugars up, so eat regularly and enjoy some healthy snacks; eating often can also help reduce nausea. I know it's tempting to reach into the cookie jar, and of course this is fine every so often, but it won't make you feel better in the long run. Have a look at the Healthy Snacks and Sweet Treats chapters for some ideas (see pages 168–203).

Some women, however, find that they have lost their appetite completely and the sheer sight and smell of food is enough to make them run a mile. If that sounds like you, please don't worry. You can rest assured that if you have had a balanced and healthy diet before falling pregnant (hopefully through eating from the preconception chapter!) then you will have laid down a healthy supply of the essential minerals and vitamins for when you need them.

This is also a good opportunity to get your partner involved – after all, it takes two to tango; get them behind the stove if you really can't face it. Little and often is my tip during the first 12 weeks. Bulk cooking is also great, so that you have something good to eat when you really don't feeling like getting the chopping board out.

Whatever your preferences and however you are feeling, there is plenty to suit you in this chapter.

Baby's Development In The First Trimester: 0–12 Weeks

Major nutrients needed during the first 12 weeks of development are: protein, vitamins A, B6, B12, C and D, beta-carotene, essential fatty acids (DHA, see page 9), folate, iron, zinc, calcium, magnesium and selenium.

During the first 12 weeks of pregnancy your baby will grow the fastest that it will throughout the whole pregnancy. By the end of week 12, all of your baby's organs will be formed and it will resemble a human. Its arms and legs grow rapidly, along with muscles that begin to develop. For this to happen we need to be eating foods rich in calcium, protein and carbohydrates.

Your baby's central nervous system starts to develop and become ready to mature. The B-group vitamins will play a strong role here, along with protein, zinc, folate and calcium.

Your baby's heart will start beating for the first time and its blood will start to circulate. To do this, your baby will absorb protein, B vitamins, iron, folate, calcium and zinc from you.

As your baby's brain and muscles form and grow, calcium, B vitamins, potassium and essential fatty acids will help baby's bones start to form and harden. Your baby will also absorb magnesium, zinc, protein and vitamin C to help with this.

Your baby's eyes develop in the first eight weeks of pregnancy, although it will not be able to sense light for quite some time. Vitamins A, B2 and D, and beta-carotene are all essential for healthy eyesight in your baby.

Skin, hair and ears also start to form with the help of selenium and vitamins A, B and D.

STRAWBERRY COMPOTE AND YOGURT RIPPLE

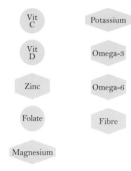

Vit C

Potassium

Vit D

Omega-3

Zinc

Omega-6

Folate

Fibre

Magnesium

Fruit compotes are great with yogurt and to have on porridge, in smoothies, on cereals or on top of ice cream when you want a treat. You can make them with most fruits but I have chosen strawberries here, not only because they have just come into season as I am writing this chapter, but also because they are a great source of vitamin C, which increases the absorption rate of iron and, in turn, helps prevent anaemia. Flaxseed is a great source of omega-3, believed to be essential for your growing baby's eye and brain development, so get sprinkling!

PREP TIME 15 MINUTES • COOK TIME 10 MINUTES • MAKES 10 PORTIONS

FOR THE COMPOTE
1kg strawberries, hulled
   (cut very large ones
   into quarters)
1 vanilla pod, split
   lengthways
3 cardamom pods
juice of 2 lemons
100ml agave nectar

TO SERVE
100ml natural yogurt
2 tbsp strawberry compote
1 tsp milled flaxseed
1 tsp sunflower seeds
1 tsp Brazil nuts, chopped

1 Sterilise a 1 litre Kilner jar or 3 x 300ml jam jars – see the instructions on page 37 for sterilising jars.

2 Place the strawberries in a large saucepan with the vanilla pod, lightly crushed cardamom pods, lemon juice and agave nectar. Slowly simmer over a low heat, stirring frequently, until the compote is the consistency you prefer. I like mine chunky so I usually simmer it for 10 minutes, but you can cook yours for longer if you prefer a softer texture.

3 Spoon the compote into your sterilised jar(s) along with the vanilla pod and cardamom, as the spices will continue to infuse into the compote in the jar. Store in the fridge for up to 2 weeks once opened. (If stored properly in a sealed jar it can keep for up to a year.)

4 To serve, pour the yogurt into a tumbler or bowl, add a couple of tablespoons of strawberry compote and gently ripple it through. Sprinkle with the seeds and nuts before eating. Alternatively, you could scatter some Healthy Flaxseed and Fig Granola over the top (see opposite).

HEALTHY FLAXSEED AND FIG GRANOLA

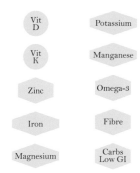

Vit D

Vit K

Zinc

Iron

Magnesium

Potassium

Manganese

Omega-3

Fibre

Carbs Low GI

I know there are loads of different types of granola on the supermarket shelves, but by making your own you know exactly what has gone into it and therefore exactly what and how much goodness you are eating. This granola recipe is great both for preconception and throughout your pregnancy. It contains plant proteins as well as omega-3 to make for a very healthy body and mind. I make my granola in a big batch, which lasts for a couple of weeks, and I vary what I put in it from time to time.

PREP TIME 10 MINUTES • COOK TIME 30 MINUTES • MAKES 800G (8–10 PORTIONS)

75g Brazil nuts
75g pecans
75g dried figs, dates
    or apricots
300g rolled oats
50g milled flaxseed
100g pumpkin seeds
100g sunflower seeds
50g flaked almonds
2 tsp ground cinnamon
3 tbsp runny honey
2 tbsp rapeseed oil

1 Preheat the oven to 170°C (fan 150°C) and line a baking tray with parchment.

2 Place the Brazil nuts, pecans and dried fruit into a food processor and pulse 6–8 times until they are roughly chopped. Add all the remaining ingredients and pulse again 3–4 times to combine everything together well.

3 Sprinkle the mixture on to the lined baking tray and cook in the oven for 20–30 minutes or until slightly golden brown. Leave to cool before transferring into a 1 litre Kilner jar or airtight container, ready to serve for your delicious breakfast. The granola will stay fresh for up to 1 month.

> **SERVING SUGGESTIONS:**
>
> Almond milk, hazelnut milk or cows' milk
>
> Natural unsweetened yogurt or Greek yogurt
>
> Fresh berries, pomegranate seeds or chopped-up fruit of your choice
>
> Dried cranberries, blueberries or goji berries
>
> Manuka or any other good quality runny honey

BUCKWHEAT PANCAKES WITH BLUEBERRY COMPOTE

Vit B6

Vit B2

Vit C

Manganese

Folate

Calcium

Fibre

Make a big batch of these at the weekend for brunch, when you have a little more time to relax, then freeze the leftovers for when you don't have time to cook or are feeling too unwell to do so. Simply freeze any pancakes you don't eat between sheets of greaseproof paper and store in a freezer-safe container, then heat one or two in the microwave or a hot pan with a little butter when you feel the need for a hearty breakfast – they will taste just as delicious.

Buckwheat contains slow-releasing and nourishing carbohydrates which will keep you feeling fuller for longer and keep any waves of sickness at bay. Blueberries are rich in vitamin C, which will help contribute towards a healthy immune system, essential for you and your developing embryo. I buy blueberries in large batches when they are in season, from June to September, and freeze them whole or make lots of compote to freeze.

PREP TIME 10 MINUTES • COOK TIME 20 MINUTES • MAKES 8–10

225g buckwheat flour
2 tsp ground cinnamon
2 tsp baking powder
2 free-range eggs
225ml almond milk or
　semi-skimmed cows' milk
2 tbsp maple syrup
2 tbsp butter, melted
2–3 tbsp rapeseed oil

FOR THE COMPOTE
400g blueberries, fresh
　or frozen
1 tsp vanilla bean paste
2 tbsp agave nectar
　or maple syrup

TO SERVE
natural yogurt
maple syrup (optional)

1 Make the pancake batter by sifting the buckwheat flour, cinnamon and baking powder into a bowl. Make a well in the centre and crack in the eggs. Beat the eggs, bringing in some of the flour from the sides of the bowl to form a paste. Add half the milk and mix again, whisking in the remaining flour as you mix. When you have a smooth, thick paste, beat in the rest of the milk, the maple syrup and the melted butter. Leave the batter to rest while you make the compote.

2 Place the blueberries in a small saucepan over a low heat and add the vanilla bean paste and agave nectar. Cook for 5–10 minutes, until the berries burst, stirring once or twice so they don't catch on the bottom of the saucepan. Turn off the heat and leave to cool slightly.

3 Heat a large frying pan over a medium heat, add 1 tablespoon of rapeseed oil and wipe it around the pan using kitchen roll. Pour half a ladle of pancake batter into the pan. You should be able to cook 2–3 pancakes at a time, depending on the size of your frying pan. Turn the pancakes over when bubbles start to appear on the surface of the batter, after about 2 minutes. Cook until golden brown on both sides. Repeat this process, adding a little more oil each time, until you have used all the batter.

4 Serve the pancakes with a large spoonful of compote and a dollop of yogurt. Drizzle over more maple syrup if you fancy it.

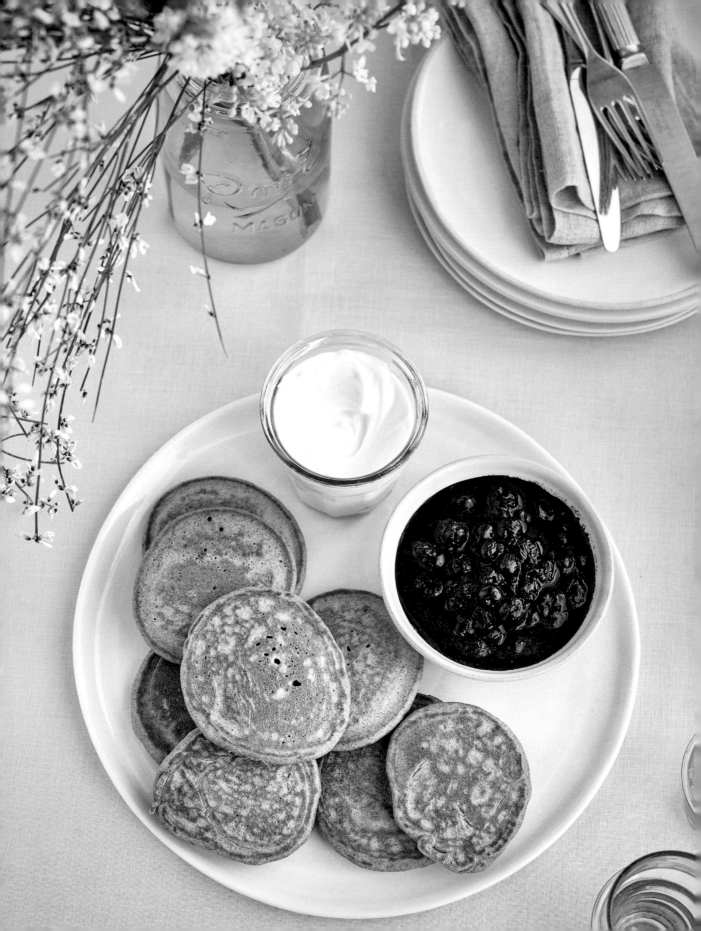

FETA AND TOMATO PAN-BAKED EGGS

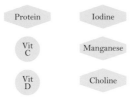

Protein · Iodine · Vit C · Manganese · Vit D · Choline

Eggs contain iodine, which is essential for the healthy development of your baby's nervous system, especially in the first three months. I ate this dish a lot in my first trimester. I found that baked eggs, rather than scrambled, were easy to digest and helped settle my stomach, not to mention being a good way to eat them when you can't have runny yolks. I was a sucker for all things salty, so feta was a great way to satisfy this craving. Tomatoes contain lots of vitamin C, which not only gives you energy but also keeps your immune system firing on all cylinders, making sure you and your baby stay healthy during these tough first three months.

PREP TIME 5 MINUTES • COOK TIME 15–20 MINUTES • SERVES 2

4 free-range eggs
2 tbsp rapeseed oil
12 baby plum
    tomatoes, halved
75g pasteurised feta
    cheese, crumbled
1 handful of watercress,
    roughly chopped
salt and freshly ground
    black pepper

TO SERVE
4 slices of rye bread
    or Super Seed Soda
    Bread (page 46)
butter

1 Preheat the grill to high. Crack the eggs into a bowl and whisk well.

2 Place a medium-sized non-stick ovenproof frying pan over a medium heat and add the rapeseed oil. Once hot, add the tomatoes. Fry them for 4–6 minutes, until they start to burst, then add the eggs. Stir well, add the feta and watercress, and season with a little salt and lots of black pepper.

3 Turn down the heat and cook on the stove for 3–5 minutes, until the eggs to start to set. Transfer the pan to the grill and cook for a further 10 minutes, to allow the dish to cook through. You need to do this or the bottom will be overcooked and the top undercooked.

4 Remove the pan from the grill, turn the baked eggs out on to a plate and enjoy with hot buttered toast.

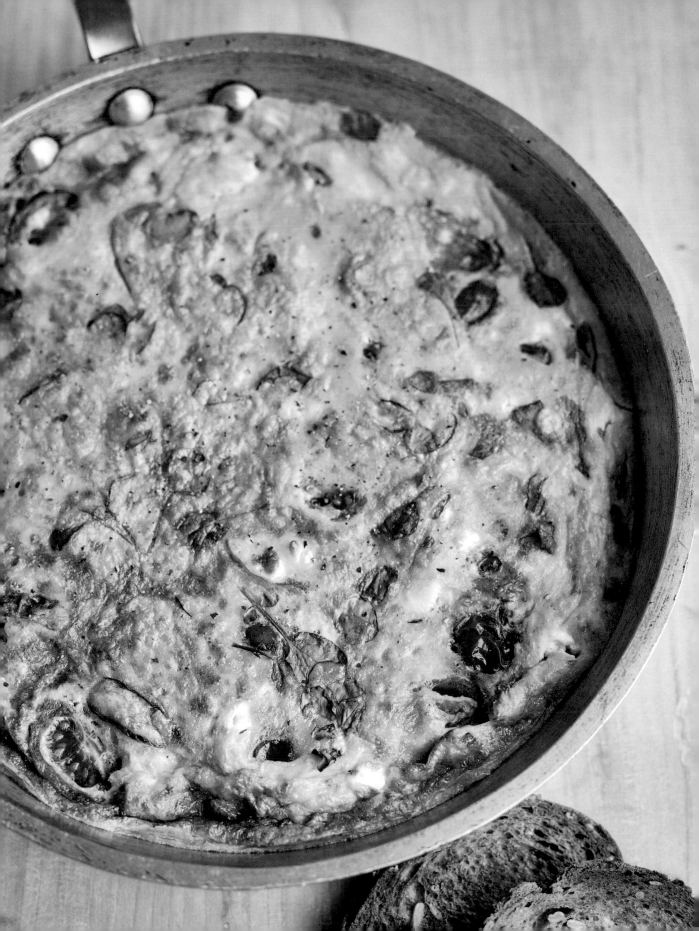

ROASTED TOMATOES ON RYE WITH AVOCADO

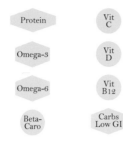

Protein

Omega-3

Omega-6

Beta-Caro

Vit C

Vit D

Vit B12

Carbs Low GI

This recipe may sound a bit simple (which if you feel like I did in the first couple of months is a blessing), but it is really good for you and your developing baby. Buy a good quality avocado or hemp seed oil to drizzle over the top and it will keep you going all morning. I had this all the time in my first trimester and it really helped set me up for the day without leaving me feeling overly full. Essential fatty acids found in hemp seed oil and avocados are essential for healthy eye and brain development in your baby.

PREP TIME 10 MINUTES • COOK TIME 10 MINUTES • SERVES 2

10 baby plum tomatoes
1 tbsp olive oil
1 ripe avocado
4 tbsp cottage cheese
zest and juice of ½ lemon
4 slices of rye bread
    or Super Seed Soda
    Bread (page 46)
1 tbsp sunflower seeds
1 tbsp pumpkin seeds
2–3 tsp avocado or hemp
    seed oil
salt and freshly ground
    black pepper

1 Preheat the oven to 220°C (fan 200°C). Place the tomatoes in a small baking dish and drizzle with the olive oil. Roast the tomatoes in the oven for 10 minutes, until they start to burst.

2 Meanwhile, cut the avocado in half and remove the stone. Scoop out the flesh using a spoon, place in a bowl and mash with the back of a fork. Season with a small amount of salt and black pepper, and fold in the cottage cheese. Mix through the lemon juice.

3 Toast the bread, then pile the cottage cheese and avocado mixture on top. Grate over the lemon zest, then scatter over the sunflower and pumpkin seeds. Top with the roasted tomatoes and drizzle with avocado or hemp seed oil.

BROCCOLI, ALMOND, CHILLI AND LEMON WHOLEWHEAT FUSILLI

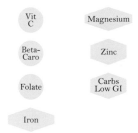

Vit C
Magnesium
Beta-Caro
Zinc
Folate
Carbs Low GI
Iron

Broccoli is a superfood for all expectant mums as it is high in folate, essential for a healthy nervous system in baby, and full of iron, which is needed for healthy red blood cells that carry oxygen around your body as well as to the placenta for baby. Wholewheat pasta is far higher in fibre than white pasta, helping you to maintain a healthy digestive system that tends to slow down during pregnancy. Use any shape you like!

PREP TIME 20 MINUTES • COOK TIME 20 MINUTES • SERVES 4

1 broccoli head, cut into florets, stalk chopped
500g wholewheat fusilli pasta
4–5 tbsp extra virgin olive oil or extra virgin rapeseed oil
4 anchovy fillets
2 garlic cloves, peeled and sliced
1–2 pinches of dried red chilli
1 tbsp Dijon mustard
juice of 1 lemon
3 tbsp flaked almonds, toasted
2 tbsp walnut oil
salt and freshly ground black pepper

FOR THE BREADCRUMBS
2 tbsp extra virgin olive oil or extra virgin rapeseed oil
4 tbsp dried breadcrumbs
2 tbsp flat-leaf parsley, finely chopped
zest of 2 lemons
salt and freshly ground black pepper

TO SERVE
30g Parmesan cheese, grated

1 Start by preparing the breadcrumbs. Heat the oil in a frying pan over a medium heat. When hot, add the breadcrumbs and stir. Allow them to toast for 5–6 minutes, until golden brown. Turn off the heat and mix through the parsley and lemon zest and season, with a little salt and pepper.

2 Cook the broccoli in a saucepan of boiling salted water for 2 minutes, until tender, then drain well. In a separate pan, cook the pasta according to the packet instructions.

3 While the pasta is cooking, set a sauté pan over a medium heat and add 2 tablespoons of the oil, the anchovies, garlic and chilli. Fry for 2 minutes before adding in the cooked broccoli. Now add the remaining oil, Dijon mustard and lemon juice. Season with salt and pepper. Remove the pan from the heat while the pasta finishes cooking.

4 When the pasta is cooked, add it to the broccoli mixture along with the flaked almonds and walnut oil. Serve with the breadcrumbs and Parmesan sprinkled over the top.

BARLEY RISOTTO WITH EMERALD PESTO AND ASPARAGUS

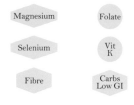

You will find a number of pulses and grains substituted for some or all of the rice in my 'risottos' throughout this book. Not only because I really do enjoy their texture and flavour, but also because they are a source of minerals, vitamins and fibre that your body simply can't do without while carrying your precious little one, and any opportunity to eat them is a good one.

PREP TIME 15 MINUTES • COOK TIME 40–50 MINUTES • SERVES 2

800ml chicken or
    vegetable stock
2 tbsp rapeseed oil
2 shallots, peeled and
    finely diced
1 celery stick, finely diced
1 leek, trimmed and
    finely diced
75g pearl barley
75g Arborio rice
12 asparagus spears,
    stalks chopped and
    tips left whole
zest of 1 lemon
2 tbsp mascarpone cheese
salt and freshly ground
    black pepper

FOR THE EMERALD
PESTO
50g hazelnuts, walnuts
    or almonds, preferably
    skin on
100g baby leaf spinach
30g flat-leaf parsley
2 garlic cloves, peeled
    and roughly chopped
zest and juice of 2 lemons
30g Parmesan cheese
150ml walnut or hazelnut oil

1 First make the pesto by blitzing all the ingredients in a mini-blender until you have a rough paste. Add a little water if you feel it's too thick and not blending.

2 Heat the stock in a saucepan on the stove until it is boiling, then turn it right down to a gentle simmer.

3 Place a large casserole or sauté pan over a medium heat and add the rapeseed oil. When hot, add the shallots, celery and leek, cover with a lid and cook for 5–6 minutes, stirring every now and then.

4 Once the vegetables are soft and translucent, add the pearl barley and cook for 2 minutes until it is coated in the oil from the pan and it starts to toast slightly. Add half of the stock and leave to simmer for 12 minutes, stirring occasionally.

5 Pour in the Arborio rice and half of the remaining stock, and increase the heat. You now need to keep stirring the risotto until all the liquid has been absorbed by the barley and rice. When it has, add the remaining stock and continue to stir until the liquid is absorbed – this should take around 15 minutes over a high heat.

6 Now add in the asparagus stalks and tips and cook for another 5 minutes, until tender.

7 When you are happy your risotto is cooked (it should have a slight bite to it), stir in all of the pesto and lemon zest and mix well. Check for seasoning; you will probably need pepper and perhaps a little salt.

8 Serve your risotto with the mascarpone on top, so that it melts in as you eat it.

ROASTED MACKEREL WITH GINGER AND CARROT SALAD

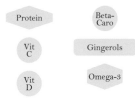

This is a really refreshing and light salad that contains lots of ginger, which should help with nausea and digestion. Ginger is also antibacterial, so will help keep your immune system good and strong. The carrots contain lots of beta-carotene, which supports protection against eye defects, and the mackerel will provide you with all the omega-3 your body requires for that day, which in turn will help support the development of baby's brain and eye development and is also needed for the absorption of essential vitamins A, D, E and K.

PREP TIME 15 MINUTES • COOK TIME 12 MINUTES • SERVES 2

2 x 125g fresh mackerel
   fillets, pin-boned, skin on
2 tbsp rapeseed oil
juice of 1 lime
2 tbsp soy sauce

FOR THE SALAD
5cm piece fresh ginger,
   peeled and grated
zest and juice of 2 limes
1 tsp runny honey or
   agave nectar
1 red chilli, deseeded
   and chopped (optional)
400g carrots, peeled
   and grated
15g fresh mint or coriander
   leaves, roughly chopped
2 tbsp plain peanuts,
   toasted and crushed
salt

1 Preheat the oven to 200°C (fan 180°C). Season the mackerel fillets with the rapeseed oil, lime juice and soy sauce. Place on a baking tray and roast in the oven for 12 minutes.

2 While the mackerel is cooking, make the salad. Mix the ginger with the lime zest and juice, honey and chilli, if using, and a generous pinch of salt. Pour this dressing over the grated carrot in a bowl and stir in before adding the herbs and peanuts.

3 Lay the cooked fish on top of the salad and enjoy while warm. This is also great cold the next day for lunch – reserve a few fresh herbs to mix through before eating.

KALE, RED QUINOA AND ROASTED SQUASH SALAD WITH TOASTED SEEDS

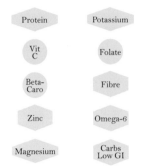

Protein · Potassium · Vit C · Folate · Beta-Caro · Fibre · Zinc · Omega-6 · Magnesium · Carbs Low GI

I often make this salad with Puy lentils rather than quinoa and both options are equally tasty. Quinoa is a grain-like seed that cooks quickly and is really very good for you. It will fill you up and provide you with lots of protein, which equals energy for mum and growing baby. Kale is a superfood in its own right. Rich in iron, it is a food we must eat to keep iron levels up and reduce the risk of anaemia. The seeds in this dish will also help bolster iron levels.

PREP TIME 15 MINUTES • COOK TIME 15 MINUTES • SERVES 2

½ small butternut squash, deseeded and cut into 2cm cubes (no need to peel)
1 tsp ground ginger
½ tsp dried chilli flakes
2 tsp paprika
3 tbsp rapeseed oil
1 tbsp runny honey
50g red quinoa, washed
150g green or purple kale
75g pasteurised feta cheese
2–3 tbsp mixed seeds (e.g. sunflower, pumpkin, sesame, poppy seeds), toasted
salt and freshly ground black pepper

FOR THE DRESSING
5cm piece fresh ginger, peeled and grated
zest and juice of 1 lemon
1 tbsp runny honey
1 tsp Dijon mustard
3–4 tbsp walnut oil

1 Preheat the oven to 200°C (fan 180°C). Place the butternut squash in a bowl. Stir in the ginger, chilli flakes, paprika, and salt and pepper, and drizzle with the rapeseed oil and honey. Line a baking sheet with parchment. Spread the coated butternut squash out on the parchment and roast in the oven for 15 minutes.

2 While the squash is cooking, prepare the rest of the salad. Cook the quinoa in a saucepan of boiling salted water for 12 minutes or until tender. Drain, then tip into a bowl and set aside. Blanch the kale in a separate pan of salted boiling water; cook for 1 minute before draining and running under cold water to stop it overcooking.

3 Make the dressing by putting all the ingredients in a small jar, placing the lid on and shaking hard until everything is well combined.

4 Once the squash is cooked, mix it into the warm quinoa and fold in the kale. Crumble in the feta cheese, sprinkle over the seeds and pour over all of the dressing. Mix and season well with salt and pepper before serving.

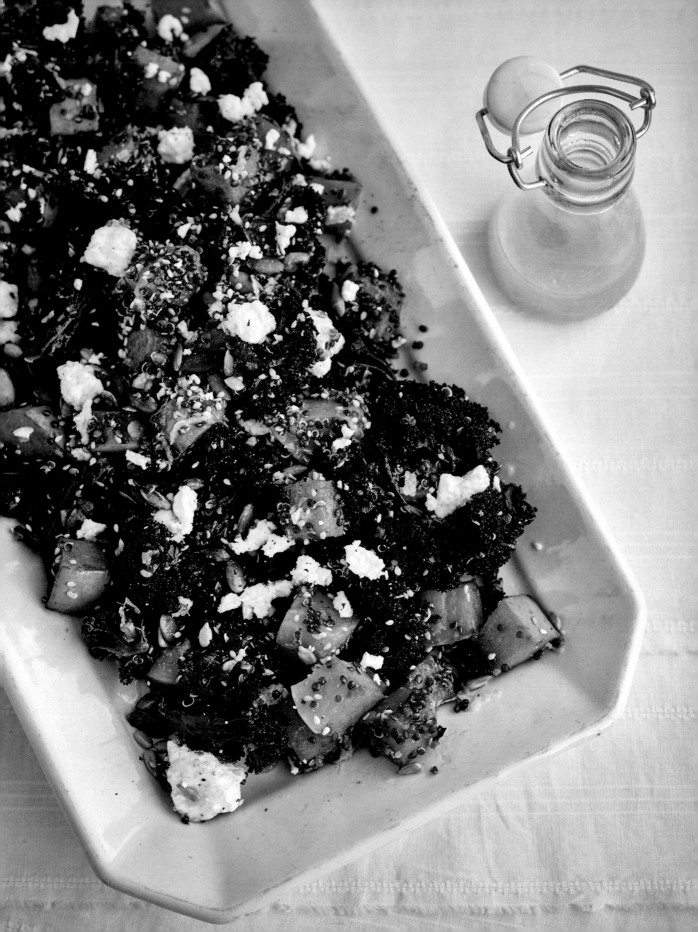

POACHED CHICKEN WITH GINGER AND LEMONGRASS BROTH

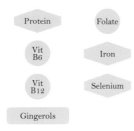

Protein
Folate
Vit B6
Iron
Vit B12
Selenium
Gingerols

A simply flavoured light broth is just the thing when you feel like you need a little bit of healing from the inside out. I have kept this recipe as simple and plain as possible – it's great if you don't have a huge appetite during the first trimester. The ginger should go some way to helping relieve symptoms of nausea, as will the delicate healing broth, which will keep you hydrated. Feel free to add other ingredients if you like, such as green beans, spring onions or mint, and for something more substantial throw in some soba noodles.

PREP TIME 20 MINUTES • COOK TIME 1 ¾ HOURS • SERVES 4

1 x 1–1.2kg free-range chicken
1 leek, trimmed and thickly sliced
1 white onion, peeled and sliced
2 carrots, peeled and thickly sliced
1 garlic bulb, cut in half crosswise
1 lemongrass stick, squashed with the back of a knife
5cm piece fresh ginger, peeled and sliced
salt and freshly ground black pepper

FOR THE FINISHED BROTH
6cm piece fresh ginger, peeled and cut into matchsticks
2 carrots, peeled and cut into matchsticks
1 handful of bean sprouts

TO SERVE (OPTIONAL)
fresh coriander leaves
alfalfa sprouts
radish sprouts

1 Place the chicken in a large casserole pan and add all the other ingredients for the broth. Cover completely with cold water, season generously with salt and bring to the boil. Once boiling, turn the heat down and allow to simmer, covered with a lid, for 1¼ hours.

2 Once the chicken is cooked, turn off the heat. Remove the chicken from the stock and place it on a plate. Set a sieve over a large clean saucepan and pour the broth through it. The cooked vegetables and aromatics have now done their job and can be discarded or blitzed into a vegetable soup (minus the garlic, lemongrass and ginger).

3 Shred the chicken meat into bite-sized pieces and add it to the strained broth. (You may not need all of it, and can keep some back for a chicken salad.) Add the strips of ginger and simmer for 4–5 minutes to heat through. Check for seasoning.

4 Place the raw carrot and bean sprouts in the bottom of your serving bowls and ladle the hot stock and chicken over the top. Serve steaming hot and sprinkle over some fresh coriander, and alfalfa and radish sprouts, if you like.

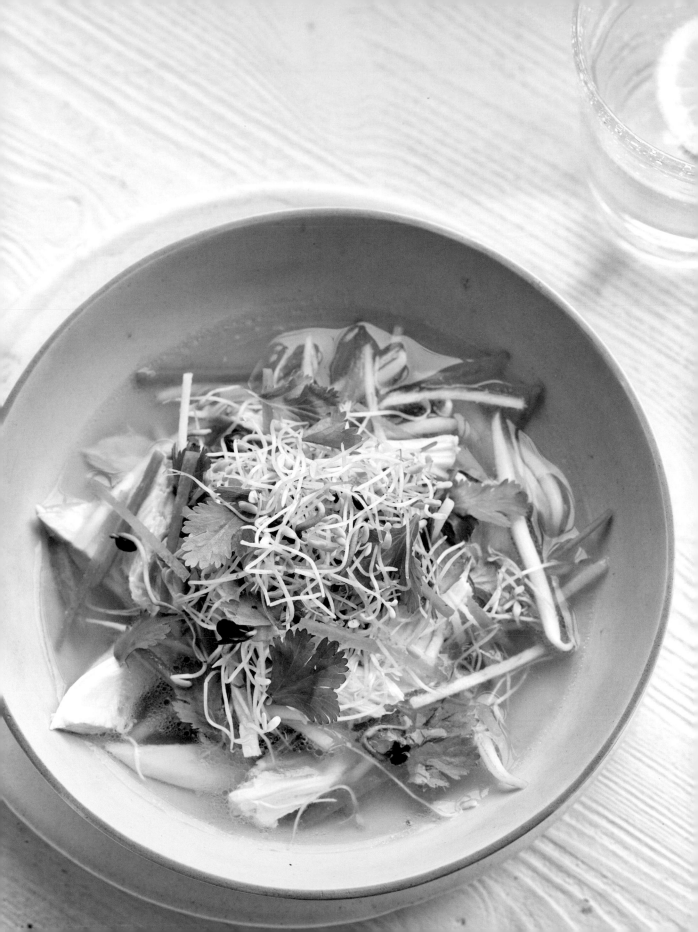

HEALTHY CHICKEN AND SWEET POTATO CHIPS

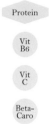

Protein

Vit B6

Vit C

Beta-Caro

Pregnancy is very subjective, and every woman has different experiences with regard to what they fancy eating and when. I've spoken to many women about what they craved during the first trimester of pregnancy. Many, like me, needed to feel full and overload on carbohydrates, while others had no appetite at all and found that only small meals of plain wholesome food would help keep the sickness at bay. This recipe is for the first group. I felt constantly hungry during the first trimester and this recipe was something I cooked many times.

PREP TIME 30 MINUTES • COOK TIME 25 MINUTES • SERVES 2

100ml buttermilk
2 x 120–150g free-range
  skinless chicken breasts,
  or turkey breast steaks
2 slices wholemeal bread
  (stale is best, or dried out
  in the oven)
50g bran flakes
2 tbsp flat-leaf parsley,
  finely chopped
salt and freshly ground
  black pepper

FOR THE SWEET
  POTATO CHIPS
2 large sweet potatoes
2 tbsp rapeseed oil
1 tsp smoked paprika
1 tsp ground cumin
1 tsp dried oregano
salt and freshly ground
  black pepper

TO SERVE
2 lemon wedges
salt

1 Preheat the oven to 200°C (fan 180°C). Pour the buttermilk into a large bowl and season with salt and pepper. Butterfly the chicken breasts by slicing them almost all of the way through the middle crossways and opening them out like a book. (If you are using turkey, put the steaks between two sheets of cling film and bash them with a rolling pin to flatten them to around ½cm thick.) Marinate the chicken in the buttermilk for 20 minutes to tenderise it.

2 Meanwhile, prepare the sweet potatoes by cutting them into 3cm-thick chips and place them in a bowl. Leave the skin on, as it not only tastes delicious but will also stop the chips falling apart during cooking. Add the remaining ingredients for the chips and mix well to coat thoroughly. Line a tray with baking parchment and spread the seasoned chips on it.

3 Blitz the stale bread with the bran flakes until they are fine crumbs, then add in the parsley. Remove the chicken from the buttermilk and coat well in the crumb mixture.

4 Place the chicken on the tray with the chips and cook in the oven for 10 minutes. Remove the tray from the oven, turn over the chips and chicken breasts, and cook for another 15 minutes.

5 The chips should now be nice and crispy and the chicken coating crisp and golden brown. Remove from the oven and serve with a wedge of lemon and a sprinkle of salt.

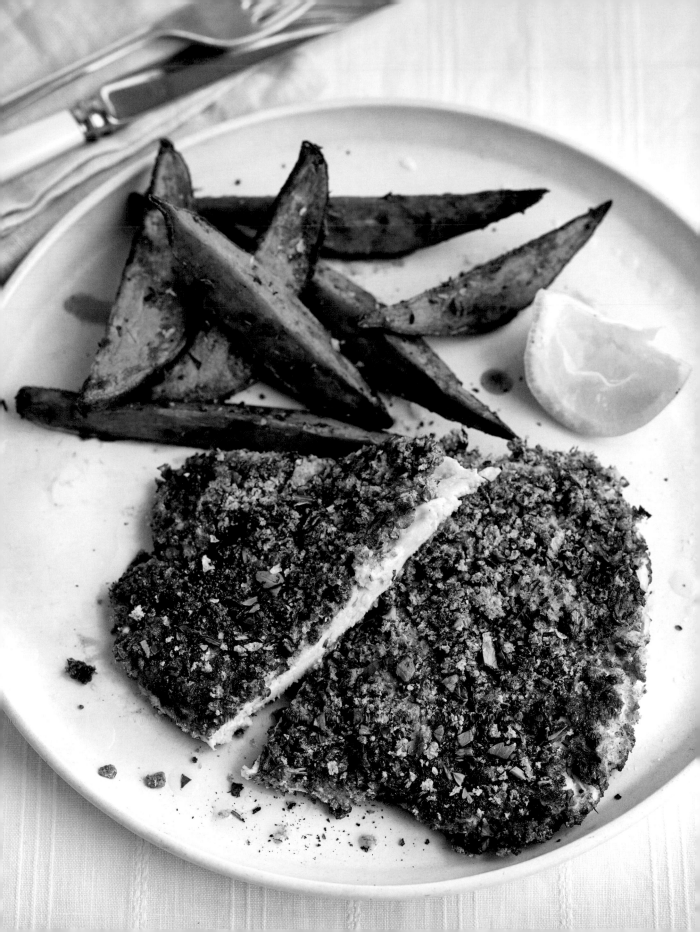

ROASTED PORK WITH PEARS AND FENNEL SEEDS

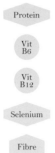

Protein

Vit B6

Vit B12

Selenium

Fibre

Pork is rich in selenium, which needs to be present in your diet to help with the development and growth of baby's ears, skin and eyes. Selenium is also important for your hormone balance during the testing time of the first trimester. Constipation and nausea are common complaints at this time, so the fibre from the pears will help keep things regular and your digestive system nice and healthy. Fennel seeds are often used to counteract nausea; try them crushed in some warm water during the day instead of your usual tea.

PREP TIME 10 MINUTES • COOK TIME 30 MINUTES • SERVES 2

2 pears, cored and
cut into eighths
350g baby new potatoes,
halved
2 fresh thyme sprigs,
leaves picked
2 tbsp fennel seeds
2 tbsp rapeseed oil,
plus extra to drizzle
1 tbsp runny honey
or maple syrup
1 pork fillet or tenderloin
(approx 400g)
salt and freshly ground
black pepper

1 Preheat the oven to 200°C (fan 180°C). Place the pears, potatoes, thyme leaves (reserving a few for the pork), fennel seeds, oil and honey in a large bowl, mix well and season with salt and pepper. Spread the coated pears and potatoes out on a baking tray and roast in the oven for 10 minutes.

2 Slice the pork fillet into 4 pieces and season well with salt and pepper, the reserved thyme leaves and a drizzle of oil. After the initial 10 minutes, remove the baking tray from the oven and add the pork, cut side down. Roast for a further 25 minutes until the potatoes and pears are golden brown and the pork is firm to the touch. (If you are worried that the pork won't be cooked you can check by inserting a metal skewer into the thickest part of the fillet. Leave it for 5 seconds before removing and placing the skewer on the back of your hand. If it is very hot, the pork is ready and safe to eat.)

3 Remove from the oven and set to one side to rest under a sheet of foil for 5 minutes. Slice the pork and serve with the potatoes and pears. Drizzle over any juices from the cooking tray and eat immediately.

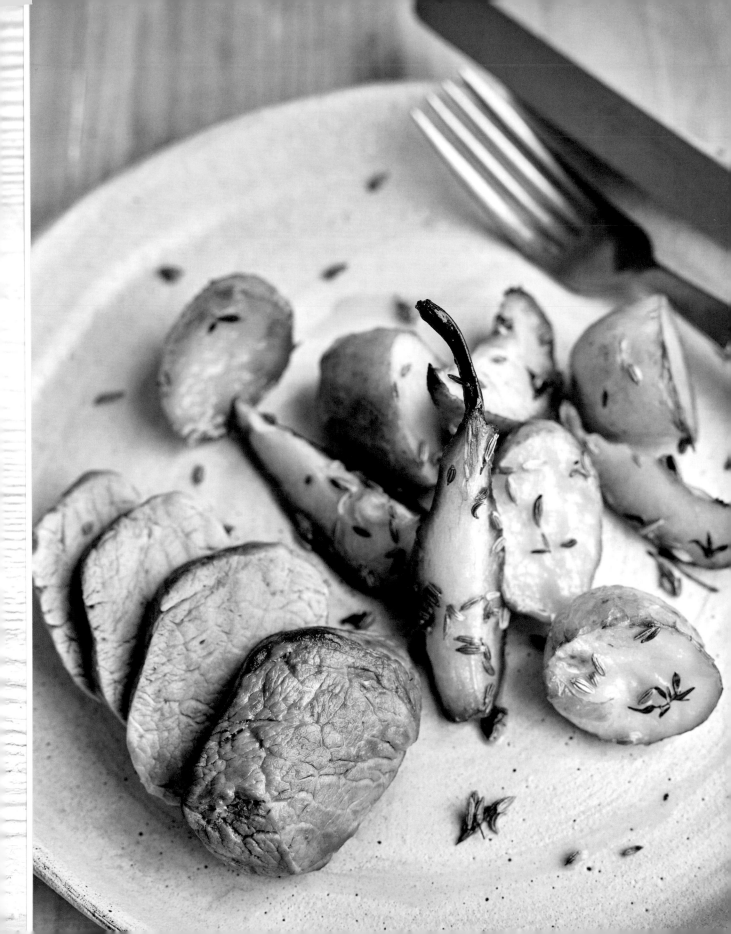

You have passed the 12-week mark! For me this was the most enjoyable part of pregnancy. Your placenta is now fully formed and your hormone levels, which peaked during the first part of your pregnancy, should start to stabilise, leaving you feeling (hopefully) a little more like your old self. Before this point, high hormone levels, blood pressure fluctuations or changes in carbohydrate metabolism can all contribute to the dreaded morning sickness – you may begin to see the back of this now and your energy levels lift. If you haven't yet started to feel the benefits of settling hormones, don't panic! Everyone is different and no pregnancy is the same. Continue to eat the recipes from the first trimester that are designed to help with morning sickness (like the Poached Chicken with Ginger and Lemongrass Broth on page 80), as well as beginning to incorporate the new recipes in this chapter into your diet if you can. Feeling bloated, tired and sick can leave you feeling a little down in the dumps, but try to remember that it won't last for ever and you will have a wonderful prize at the end of your journey.

During this second trimester, many women find they develop a bigger appetite than they had in their first trimester. It can be hard to resist unhealthy snacks like cakes and biscuits, but try to eat foods with a low glycaemic index or that contain nourishing carbohydrates (see page 12 for more information on carbohydrates and food groups, and the nutritional food chart on pages 6–11). Baby is growing rapidly at this stage and over the next three months will triple in size, so a little weight gain is perfectly normal – 1–2kg per month is about average. This is caused by the weight of your growing baby, the growing placenta and the water that baby is surrounded by. If you are worried you aren't gaining enough weight or are gaining too much, speak to your midwife, who can give you lots of information and guidance.

Try to enjoy this part of your pregnancy. Around this time, a little bump may be starting to appear and most women feel that it is safe to let people know about their little one. This is such an exciting time: if you haven't already had it, your 12-week scan is just around the corner and you will soon get your first glimpse of that tiny little bubba in your belly. I can assure you that at that stage, it will all start to feel very real indeed – you will appreciate the good wishes and support that you won't necessarily have had before now. You can also start to show off your growing and blossoming bump, and feel the benefit of all those pregnancy hormones that give you lovely glossy hair and glowing skin – not to mention the luxury of getting a seat on public transport!

Baby's Development In The Second Trimester: 13–28 Weeks

Major nutrients needed during weeks 13–28 of development are: vitamins B, C, D and E, omega-3 essential fatty acids, calcium, iron, folate, zinc, iodine and magnesium.

Your baby will grow up to three times its length in the next three months. Its muscles, skin and hair will start to grow. Protein is essential for this to happen, as well as the vitamin B family, vitamin D, zinc and magnesium. Fat will begin to cover its body and its bones will start to harden. This is why calcium is really important at this stage, along with vitamin D and magnesium.

Your baby's brain, nervous system and immune system will also begin their complex development. For this to happen our bodies will need to share omega-3, zinc, iodine, calcium, and B vitamins with the baby.

Baby's muscles and nerves connect and start to respond to the rapidly growing brain. This connection should increase the baby's movements and as it starts to grow larger and become stronger, you will begin to feel little flutters, the first feelings of your baby moving around in your womb.

By 16–18 weeks, these flutters may start to turn into stronger little kicks…and maybe the occasional punch! For some women, however, this doesn't happen until a little later on, past the 20-week stage.

PINK GRAPEFRUIT, PEACH AND PISTACHIO SALAD

Sometimes you just want something fresh and light, and this is exactly that. Peaches are an excellent source of fibre, as are pistachios. Fibre is very important while pregnant, and especially as your digestive system starts to slow down in the later weeks.

I often have this salad with a spoonful of ricotta cheese to bulk it out a bit and add some protein.

PREP TIME 5 MINUTES • SERVES 2

1 tbsp agave nectar
½ tsp orange blossom water
1 large pink grapefruit
2 large ripe white peaches (you could use tinned peaches or nectarines if fresh ones aren't in season)
10 fresh mint leaves
50g pistachio nuts, chopped

1 Pour the agave nectar and orange blossom water into a ramekin or small bowl and mix together well.

2 Top and tail the grapefruit and cut away the skin and pith using a small serrated knife. Cut the peeled grapefruit into slices or segments. Cut the peaches into eighths, discarding their stones, and mix with the grapefruit in a bowl.

3 Divide the peach and grapefruit pieces between two serving plates and pour over the agave mixture. Tear over the mint leaves and sprinkling over the chopped pistachios.

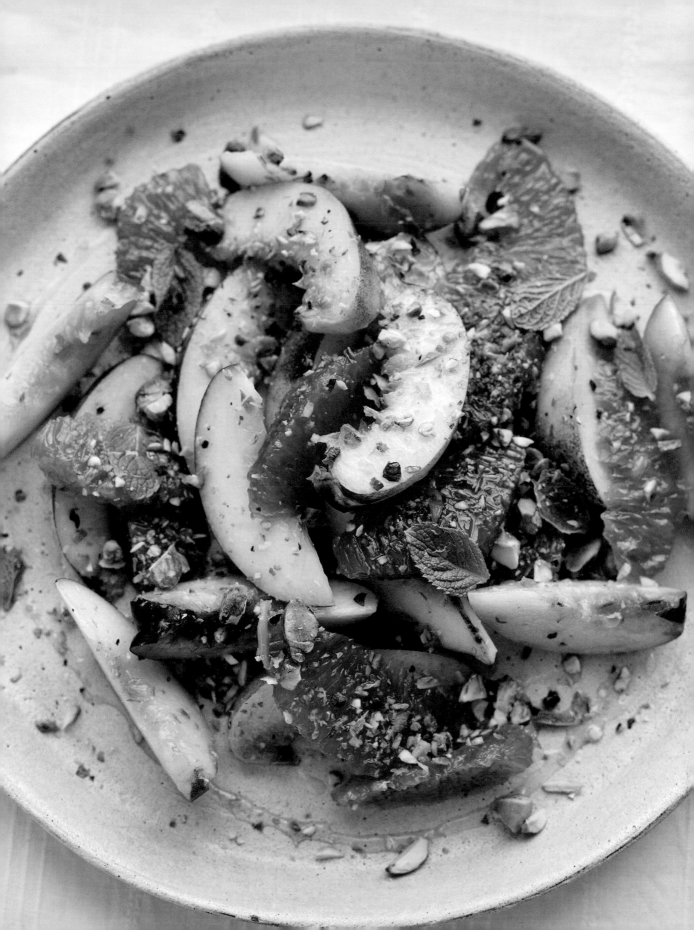

BLUEBERRY AND VANILLA RICOTTA CRÊPES

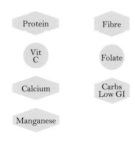

Protein

Vit C

Calcium

Manganese

Fibre

Folate

Carbs Low GI

Blueberries are packed full of vitamin C, folate and fibre – all great for building immunity and a healthy digestive system, and for boosting energy levels. Delicious raw or cooked, there is something quite special about them when cooked until just warm and wilted, so that when you bite into them they self-sauce, creating an instant mouthful of jam for whatever you pair them with. Ricotta is a fresh cheese, often made from sheeps' milk but now more commonly cows' milk, and is a very good source of calcium. It makes a great filling for crêpes, as it's wonderfully creamy without being too heavy.

PREP TIME 10 MINUTES • COOK TIME 15–20 MINUTES • MAKES 6–8

150g wholemeal flour
   or spelt flour
1 free-range egg
325ml semi-skimmed cows'
   milk or almond milk
20g butter
50ml rapeseed oil

FOR THE FILLING
200g ricotta cheese
4 tbsp runny honey
1 vanilla pod, split
   lengthways and seeds
   removed, or 1 tsp
   vanilla bean paste
zest of 1 orange

FOR THE WARM
   BLUEBERRIES
200g blueberries
2 tbsp water
1 tbsp runny honey
   or agave nectar

1 Make the crêpe batter by sifting the flour into a large bowl. Create a well in the centre, crack in the egg and pour in half of the milk. Using a whisk, mix well, incorporating the flour from the sides of the bowl bit by bit. Once you have formed a thick paste, add the remaining milk and whisk again until smooth. Leave the batter to rest while you make your filling.

2 Combine the ricotta with the honey, vanilla seeds and orange zest, and beat well.

3 Place the blueberries in a small saucepan over a low heat with the water and honey or agave nectar. Cook for 5–6 minutes until the berries start to wilt. Turn the heat off.

4 Now heat a 15cm non-stick frying pan or crêpe pan over a medium heat and add the butter. Once it has melted, whisk it into the crêpe batter.

5 Heat a little of the rapeseed oil in the same frying pan and, once hot, add a ladle of the crêpe mixture. Swirl the pan around as soon as the batter hits the hot pan to make sure the whole base of the pan is covered. Place the pan back on the heat and cook for 2 minutes before flipping the crêpe over and cooking the other side. Transfer to a plate. Cover the cooked crêpes with foil to keep them warm while you cook the rest and place some parchment in between each crêpe to prevent them from sticking together as you stack them.

6 Lay the warm crêpes out one at a time and fill with a little of the ricotta mixture before rolling up into cigars and serving with a couple of spoonfuls of the warm blueberries.

EARL GREY AND GINGER PRUNE COMPOTE

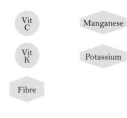

Vit C

Manganese

Vit K

Potassium

Fibre

Fibre is extremely important during pregnancy and prunes have it in abundance. Stewed prunes are great on cereal, on natural yogurt or mixed into juices and smoothies. Prunes are an excellent energy booster, and great for keeping hunger at bay during the second and third trimesters. Prunes are also a good source of vitamin K, needed for helping blood to clot properly in both you and baby.

PREP TIME 10 MINUTES • COOK TIME 20 MINUTES • MAKES 6–8 PORTIONS

2 Earl Grey tea bags (you can use decaf if you wish)
250g soft pitted prunes
5cm piece fresh ginger, peeled and finely chopped
zest and juice of 1 large orange

1 Bring 300ml of water to the boil in a small saucepan. Add the tea bags and simmer for 1 minute, then remove the tea bags and add the prunes, ginger, and orange zest and juice. Bring the mixture to the boil, then cover with a lid, reduce the heat to low and simmer for 20 minutes, until the prunes start to break down and most of the liquid has been absorbed.

2 Remove from the heat and leave the stewed prunes to cool completely.

3 Store the stewed prunes in a sterilised Kilner jar or a large jam jar – see the instructions on page 37 for sterilising jars. If stored properly in a sealed jar, the prunes will last for up to a year in the cupboard. Once opened, keep in the fridge and eat within 1 week.

4 Enjoy with some Baked Oatmeal with Banana, Pecans and Blueberries (page 98), mixed into some Chia Seed and Oat Breakfast Pots (page 47) or Healthy Flaxseed and Fig Granola (page 69), or even with a slice of Cocoa and Avocado Mousse Cake (page 194).

QUINOA BIRCHER WITH NATURAL YOGURT AND PRUNE COMPOTE

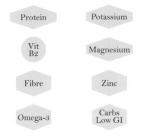

Protein

Vit B2

Fibre

Omega-3

Potassium

Magnesium

Zinc

Carbs Low GI

Bircher muesli is a great on-the-go breakfast if you have time to prepare it in advance. Quinoa and oats are brilliant sources of energy and fibre, which will help keep you going for ages. Chia seeds are able to absorb ten times their weight in water, leaving you with a full belly, and are also a good source of omega-3. This recipe is also great with fresh blueberries and runny honey if you haven't made the Earl Grey and Ginger Prune Compote from page 95.

PREP TIME 5 MINUTES, PLUS OVERNIGHT SOAKING • SERVES 2

75g quinoa flakes (available is most big supermarkets and health-food shops)
75g pinhead or rolled porridge oats
240ml semi-skimmed cows' milk or nut milk
2 tbsp chia seeds
1 tsp ground cinnamon
zest of 1 large orange
2 tbsp pistachio nuts, chopped, plus extra to serve
1 apple or pear, grated with the skin on

TO SERVE
2 tbsp natural yogurt
2 tbsp Earl Grey and Ginger Prune Compote (page 95)
1 tbsp pumpkin seeds

1 Weigh the quinoa flakes and oats into a bowl and add the milk, chia seeds, cinnamon, orange zest, pistachios and grated apple or pear. Mix well and cover tightly with cling film. Leave in the fridge overnight.

2 In the morning, when all the liquid has been absorbed, layer the bircher muesli in glasses or small bowls with the natural yogurt and prune compote. Garnish with the extra chopped pistachios and some pumpkin seeds.

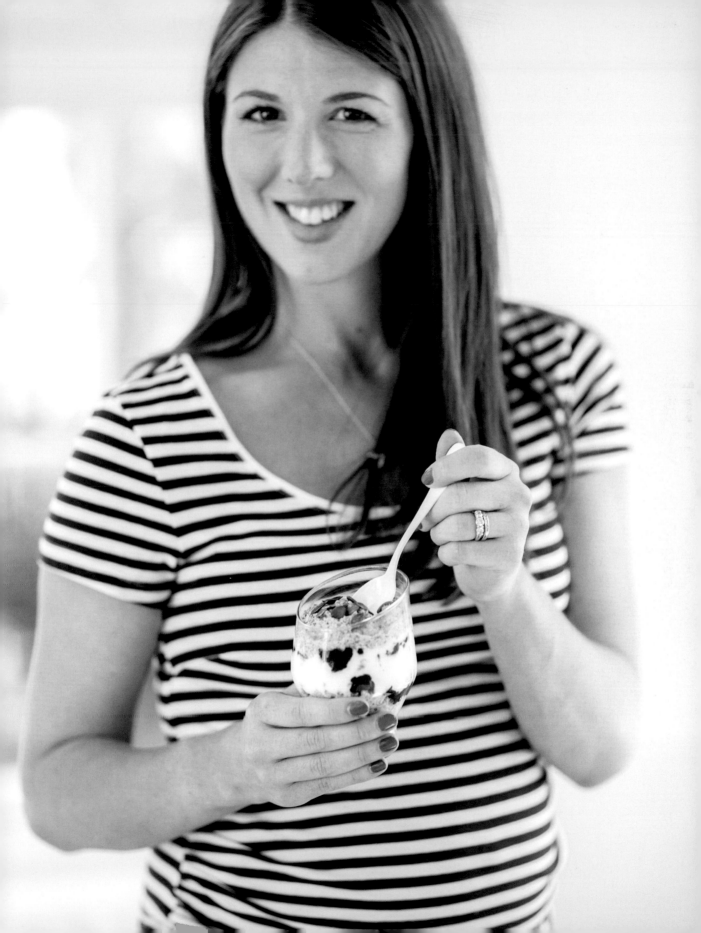

BAKED OATMEAL WITH BANANA, PECANS AND BLUEBERRIES

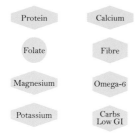

Protein
Folate
Magnesium
Potassium
Calcium
Fibre
Omega-6
Carbs Low GI

This is a fabulous weekend breakfast and one that you can put in the middle of the table and let everyone enjoy – simply multiply the quantities for more people. Baked oatmeal is completely different from porridge, although it uses pretty much the same ingredients. It has a lovely texture, with a great crispy-crunchy top once baked. This breakfast offers slow-releasing energy, so it will keep you feeling satisfied. Oats are not only great for digestion but also rich in lots of vital minerals, one of which is magnesium. Among other things, magnesium is thought to help relieve stress and anxiety during pregnancy. You may start feeling a little anxious as your pregnancy progresses, so a boost of magnesium might be just what the doctor ordered.

PREP TIME 5 MINUTES, PLUS 20 MINUTES SOAKING • COOK TIME 20 MINUTES • SERVES 2

75g rolled porridge oats
1 large banana, peeled and sliced
100g blueberries
2 tbsp runny honey
pinch of ground cloves or cinnamon
100ml semi-skimmed cows' milk or nut milk
50g pecans, chopped
1 tbsp sunflower seeds

1 Preheat the oven to 200°C (fan 180°C). Place the oats in a bowl and cover with boiling water. Leave them to soak for 20 minutes.

2 Once the oats have absorbed most of the water, drain away any excess liquid, then mix in the banana, blueberries, honey, cloves or cinnamon and the milk of your choice. Mix well before transferring to a small baking dish and sprinkling with the chopped pecans and sunflower seeds.

3 Bake in the hot oven for 15–20 minutes, until golden. Serve with some fruit compote if you have any – prune compote is especially good with baked oatmeal (see Earl Grey and Ginger Prune Compote, page 95).

EGG PAD THAI

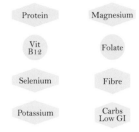

Protein · Vit B12 · Selenium · Potassium · Magnesium · Folate · Fibre · Carbs Low GI

The main ingredient in Pad Thai is the noodles. In this case they are wholewheat noodles, which are full of nourishing carbohydrates and are a good source of fibre. The eggs add essential texture, as well as being a brilliant source of protein and selenium among many other minerals and vitamins. I often add cooked chicken or prawns, or even a little bit of shredded pork left over from Sunday lunch. Leave out the chilli if you're suffering from heartburn or indigestion.

PREP TIME 20 MINUTES • COOK TIME 15 MINUTES • SERVES 2

200g wholewheat noodles
2 tbsp fish sauce
1 tbsp tamarind paste
2 tbsp crunchy
    peanut butter
1½ tbsp sweet chilli sauce
5 tbsp light soy sauce
4 tbsp rapeseed oil
4 free-range eggs, beaten
2 garlic cloves, peeled
    and finely chopped
1 red chilli, deseeded
    and sliced (optional)
4 spring onions,
    trimmed and sliced
2 large handfuls
    of bean sprouts
juice of 1 lime

TO SERVE
2 tbsp plain peanuts,
    toasted and crushed
15g fresh coriander leaves
½ red chilli, deseeded
    and sliced (optional)
2 lime wedges

1 Cook the noodles until tender in boiling salted water, according to the instructions on the packet. Once cooked, drain and leave them in cold water to stop them overcooking and sticking together.

2 In a small bowl mix together the fish sauce, tamarind paste, peanut butter, sweet chilli sauce and soy sauce. Set aside.

3 Heat half the rapeseed oil in a wok over a high heat. When hot, add the beaten eggs and scramble until well cooked. Remove from the wok into a bowl and set aside. Add the remaining oil to the wok, followed by the garlic, chilli (if using) and spring onions. Cook for a few minutes before adding the peanut butter mixture. Boil the sauce until it thickens slightly. Now drain the cooked noodles and add them to the wok, along with the cooked egg and the bean sprouts. Add the lime juice, heat through and mix well. Check for seasoning and a good balance of sweet, sour, salt and spice. If it's lacking flavour, try adding a little more lime juice or a dash more soy and fish sauce.

4 Serve the noodles with the crushed peanuts, coriander leaves, a few slices of fresh chilli and a wedge of lime.

GRILLED PRAWNS WITH PAPAYA, CASHEW AND POMEGRANATE SALAD

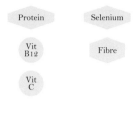

Protein

Selenium

Vit B12

Fibre

Vit C

The utterly delicious pomegranate seeds in this dish cut through the richness of the creamy cashews and juicy papaya. They freshen up the whole dish, leaving a real zing in your mouth that only pomegranates can bring. Papaya is a delicious, buttery fruit packed full of juicy goodness. It contains huge amounts of vitamin C; just what you need to allow your body to absorb iron and prevent anaemia. Vitamin C is also great for a healthy immune system, which does come under strain during pregnancy.

PREP TIME 15 MINUTES • COOK TIME 10 MINUTES • SERVES 2

10 large king prawns
2 tbsp rapeseed oil
½ tsp salt
zest and juice of 1½ limes
1 large ripe papaya
75g cashew nuts
100g pomegranate seeds
small handful of fresh
   mint leaves

1 Peel and devein the prawns. Once they are peeled (I leave the tail on for aesthetic purposes), I sometimes lay them on a chopping board and cut each prawn down its back and then open it out like a book.

2 Heat a griddle or frying pan until smoking. Sprinkle the oil and salt over the prawns, then lay them on the hot pan and cook for 5–6 minutes, turning them over halfway through, until they turn pink. Add the juice of half a lime, remove from the heat and leave to rest.

3 Cut the papaya in half and scoop out the seeds. Cut it into wedges and use a knife to cut the flesh away from the skin (like you would if cutting up a melon). Dice the flesh into small, bite-sized pieces and place in a bowl. Add to this the cashews, pomegranate seeds and the juice and zest of the other lime. Finally, shred the mint leaves and mix them through the salad.

4 Serve the grilled prawns on top of the salad. You may want to serve an extra wedge of lime on the side.

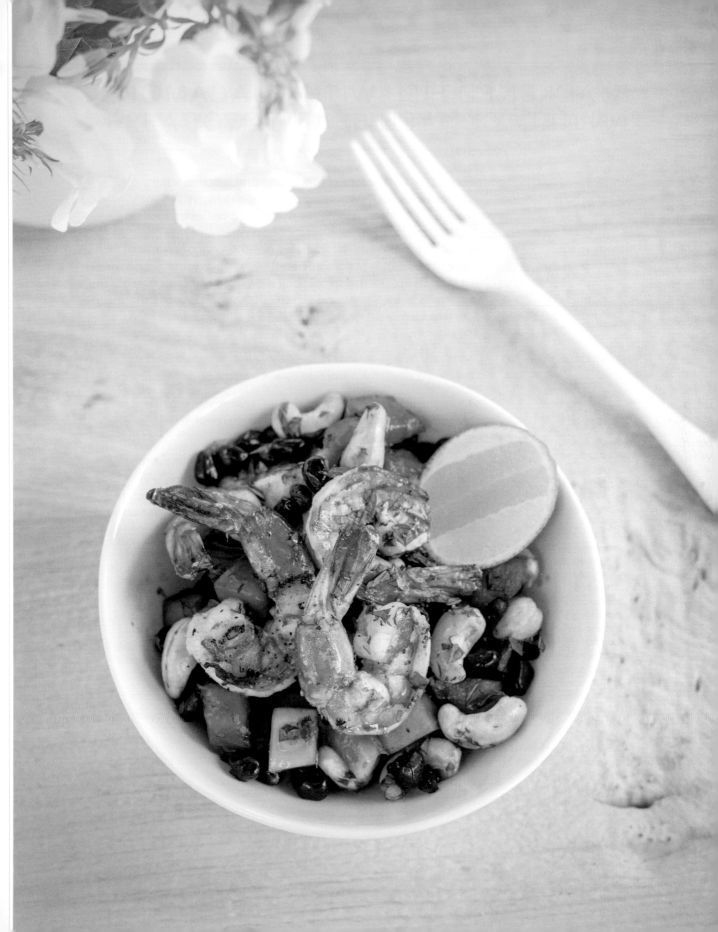

LAMB CUTLETS WITH SAFFRON, PISTACHIO AND SPINACH RICE

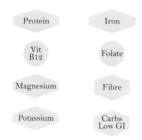

Protein	Iron
Vit B12	Folate
Magnesium	Fibre
Potassium	Carbs Low GI

I try to add extra goodness wherever I can in my recipes. In this dish, iron, folate and potassium from the pistachios will all lead the way towards a healthy pregnancy. Magnesium in the rice is essential to help baby form healthy bones and muscles. In addition, good levels of vitamin B12, found in lamb, are linked with improved mood and lower anxiety.

PREP TIME 20 MINUTES • COOK TIME 50 MINUTES • SERVES 2

6–8 lamb cutlets or chops (approx. 600–800g)
1 tsp ground cumin
1 tsp ground coriander
3 tbsp rapeseed oil
salt and freshly ground black pepper

FOR THE RICE
430ml chicken or vegetable stock
2 tbsp rapeseed oil
1 large white onion, peeled and sliced
2 garlic cloves, peeled and sliced
1 tsp ground cumin
1 tsp ground coriander
2 cardamom pods, crushed
200g brown rice
50g raisins
large pinch of saffron
50g whole pistachio nuts
2 handfuls of baby leaf spinach
salt and freshly ground black pepper

TO SERVE
2 tbsp Greek or natural yogurt
1 tbsp chopped pistachio nuts
fresh coriander leaves, torn (optional)

1 Bring the stock for the rice to the boil in a saucepan then turn off the heat.

2 Season the lamb with the cumin, coriander, salt, pepper and 1 tablespoon of the rapeseed oil. Leave to marinate while you prepare the rice.

3 Place a casserole pan on the stove, turn the heat to high and add the rapeseed oil. When hot, add the onion and fry for 2–3 minutes. Turn the heat down to medium and add the garlic, cumin, coriander and cardamom pods. Cook for 2–3 minutes before adding the rice, raisins and saffron. Cook, stirring constantly, for 1 minute to coat the rice in all the pan juices.

4 Pour in the hot stock, reserving 100ml for later. Turn the heat down to low, add a tight-fitting lid and leave to simmer for 20 minutes, stirring occasionally.

5 While the rice is cooking, set a frying pan over a high heat and pour in the remaining rapeseed oil. When hot, cook the lamb for about 3 minutes on each side, until well browned all over – do this in batches if your pan looks a little crowded, keeping the cooked chops on a warmed plate, covered with foil, while you cook the remaining ones.

6 When the rice is nearly cooked, fold in the pistachios and the spinach. Add the remaining stock, then season with salt and black pepper. Place the lamb cutlets on top and replace the lid. Leave to cook for a further 8–10 minutes until all the spinach has wilted and the liquid is absorbed.

7 Remove the lid and serve the rice and lamb. I like mine with some Greek or natural yogurt, some extra chopped pistachios and a sprinkle of torn coriander for freshness.

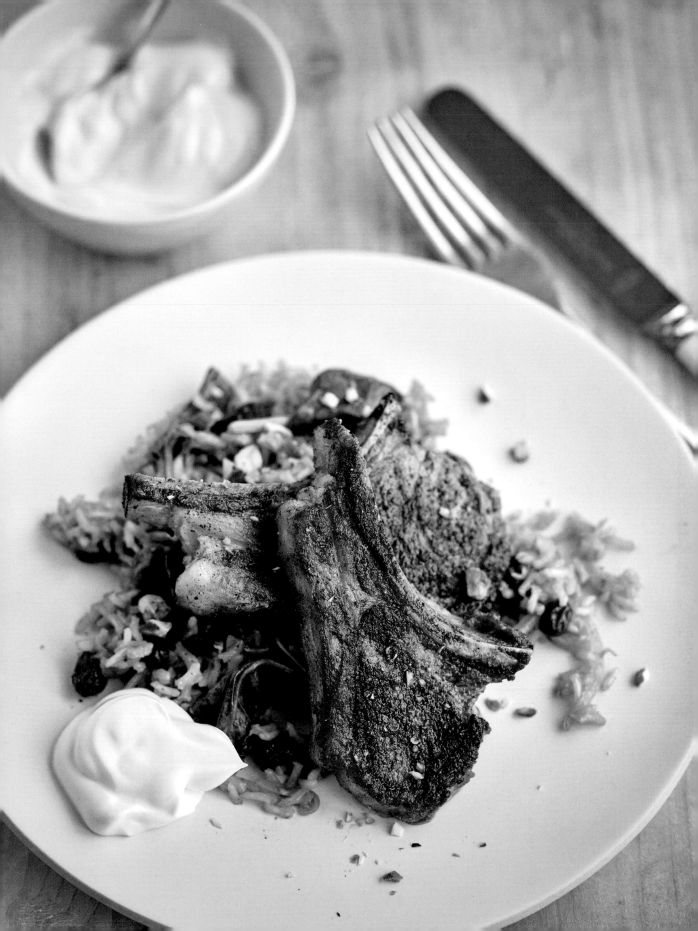

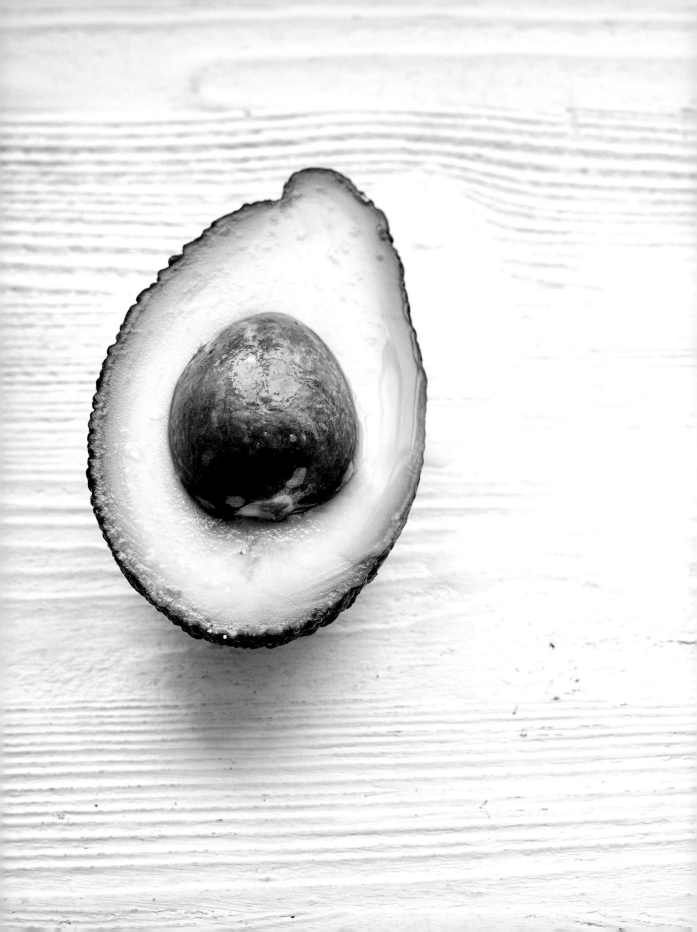

THIRD TRIMESTER

You are on the home straight; the final countdown can begin. In three months' time, you will be holding your delicious little bundle of baby. As I write this chapter, I am just starting out on my third trimester of pregnancy, 29 weeks to be exact, so I know exactly how you feel.

Energy levels will most likely be lower during this stage. In my case I'm sure that this is due to the extra weight I am carrying rather than not sleeping properly, as (for now) this seems to be OK, although my mornings do seem to be starting earlier and earlier. Leg cramps, as well as indigestion, back ache, tiredness and insomnia, are just a few of the joys we have to deal with, not to mention that, for some unlucky ladies, morning sickness and nausea might still be hanging around. Keep eating well and read back over the Food as Medicine section (pages 22–35) for some tips on how to combat some of these ailments. If troubled sleeps is one of your complaints, try a warming drink before you head off to bed. At least it will help you to relax, even if sleep is hard to come by. See pages 212–13 for some inspiration.

It is very natural to feel fed up and frustrated at times during these final few weeks – not to mention the fact that you may be starting to feel a bit nervous about the prospect of the birth, which no matter how many classes you attend and how many pregnancy books you read will seem an extremely daunting task. Believe me, I know how you feel at this particular moment as I watch my belly grow by the day! For most women, this stage of pregnancy is definitely the hardest. The waiting game can seem to go on for ever and it may start to feel like baby is never going to come out. But let's look at the positives: it's such a short time in the grand scheme of things, and soon enough you'll be holding your brand new baby in your arms and all this hard work will have been worth it.

During the final trimester of pregnancy you will need to consume a few more calories than before – not an excessive amount, just an extra 200 per day or so. Try and make sure these are made up of healthy calories that will offer extra energy and nutrients to our ever-changing bodies and to baby, who is rapidly gaining weight in the form of fat and muscle. It's really important to keep up all the good work and keep your diet well balanced, wholesome and nutritious. Try not to eat processed foods and avoid too many sweet treats if you can help it – although you definitely deserve a treat or two! See the Healthy Snacks and Sweet Treats chapters (pages 168–203) for some delicious ideas.

If you have been eating the recipes in this book, you should be noticing the benefits and your general nutritional health will be in good shape. You have been nourishing your body correctly and laying down the much-needed stores you will need to recover after the birth and during the first month or so after baby is born, especially if you are planning on breastfeeding. You have done so well so far, so don't give up on the healthy and nourishing eating now.

Baby's development in the third trimester: 29–40 Weeks

Your baby is going to be growing more rapidly than ever now and will be moving about all the time when not sleeping. Baby's position will change and it is likely to be head down in preparation for the birth. It's really important to keep up your intake of carbohydrates, protein and folate at this stage of pregnancy, to allow baby to grow to its full potential. Hair, skin and fat now cover your baby's body and it needs selenium, zinc and the vitamin B family in order to continue to produce all it needs.

Your baby's lungs will also mature, ready for its first breath in the big wide world. Calcium will be helping baby's bones and teeth to develop.

Baby's brain is constantly growing and developing, and to help with this we need to make sure that we get plenty of omega-3, zinc and iodine. These minerals, along with folate, vitamin B6 and vitamin C, will also help the nervous system and immune system begin to function, ensuring baby can fight off infection and interact properly when born.

Until now, your baby has relied on you to produce its red blood cells, but it will now start to produce its own and even lay down stores and produce its own blood. In order to do this, high amounts of iron, folate and vitamin B12 are needed.

GRATED FRUIT PORRIDGE

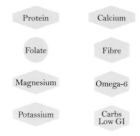

Protein

Folate

Magnesium

Potassium

Calcium

Fibre

Omega-6

Carbs
Low GI

This is a simple breakfast to make and is a really good way to start the day. It contains slow-releasing energy and complex carbohydrates, essential for maintaining energy levels and supporting the health of your rapidly growing baby. The fibre will help to get your digestive system moving and the fruit will give you instant energy, ready to start the day. Calcium and magnesium, present in the oats, may help with leg cramps and the folate will help prevent fatigue.

PREP TIME 5 MINUTES • COOK TIME 10 MINUTES • SERVES 2

100g rolled porridge oats
600ml almond or oat milk or
  semi-skimmed cows' milk
1 tsp mixed spice
4 pitted dates, chopped
1 pear, grated with the
  skin on
1 apple, grated with
  the skin on
runny honey, to taste
2 tbsp sunflower, pumpkin
  or sesame seeds,
  or milled flaxseed

1 Pour the oats into a saucepan and stir in the milk and mixed spice. Set the pan over a low heat and gently bring to the boil. Cook the porridge, stirring often, for about 5 minutes, until it is thick and creamy.

2 Add the chopped dates and cook for another 1–2 minutes before adding in the grated fruit. Stir well, add honey to taste, and serve sprinkled with the seeds.

SPELT EGGY BREAD WITH COTTAGE CHEESE AND PRUNE COMPOTE

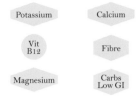

Eggy bread was one of my favourite things when I was growing up and it was always a real treat. I loved the process of soaking the bread and adding lots of lovely warm spices to the mixture, which used to make the house smell like Christmas. My nan used to make it with sliced white bread and serve it with strawberry jam or tomato ketchup for a savoury snack. I have put a twist on her very delicious but unhealthy version, creating a high-fibre and nutrient-rich alternative.

I use spelt bread, but wholegrain or rye also work really well. As a treat, you could try a spelt croissant. If you have been experiencing cramps in your legs, the potassium and magnesium in wholegrain and spelt bread should help.

PREP TIME 5 MINUTES • COOK TIME 10 MINUTES • SERVES 2

2 free-range eggs
75ml semi-skimmed
   cows' milk
pinch of ground cinnamon
1 tsp agave nectar
   or maple syrup
4 thin slices spelt bread
1 tbsp rapeseed oil
25g butter

TO SERVE
2 tbsp cream cheese
2 tbsp Earl Grey and Ginger
   Prune Compote (page 95)
1 tbsp agave nectar
   or maple syrup
2 tbsp flaked almonds

1 Heat the prune compote in a small saucepan over a low heat until the prunes are hot. Stir regularly to prevent them from sticking to the pan. You may need to add a drop of water if the consistency seems too thick. Cover to keep hot but remove from the heat.

2 Whisk the eggs with the milk, cinnamon and agave nectar or maple syrup in a large bowl. Place a large frying pan over a medium heat and add the oil. Soak the sliced bread in the eggy mixture until the bread starts to go slightly soggy. Lay your soaked sliced bread in the hot frying pan and cook for 3–4 minutes, until the bread is nicely caramelised, before turning it over and cooking the other side for the same amount of time. At this stage, add the butter to the pan and when it is foaming, spoon it all over the bread. Once cooked, remove the eggy bread from the pan on to some kitchen roll to absorb any excess oil.

3 Arrange the slices on a plate, add a spoonful of the cream cheese and top with the warm compote. Drizzle with a little more agave nectar or maple syrup and serve with a sprinkle of flaked almonds.

PORTOBELLO BAP WITH CHORIZO, WATERCRESS AND FETA

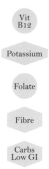

Vit B12

Potassium

Folate

Fibre

Carbs Low GI

There is nothing more satisfying in life than a big sandwich, especially at breakfast time, and this is one of my favourites. Portobello mushrooms are rich in B vitamins and potassium, both of which are extremely important in the final stages of pregnancy. Vitamin B12 helps with red blood cell formation and a healthy nervous system, and is really important for energy levels. Potassium is essential for maintaining fluid and electrolyte balance in your body, and releasing energy from proteins, fats and carbohydrates. It is also important for muscle contraction, so it's a good idea to build up your stores ready for labour. If you don't want the bread, try sandwiching the halloumi and chorizo between the cooked mushrooms – delicious.

PREP TIME 5 MINUTES • COOK TIME 10 MINUTES • SERVES 2

2 extra large portobello mushrooms, peeled
2 tbsp rapeseed oil
100g small chorizo sausages (I prefer to use the raw cooking variety)
1 garlic clove, peeled and finely chopped
juice of ½ lemon
handful of watercress
50g pasteurised feta cheese
2 wholemeal baps
salt and freshly ground black pepper

1 Drizzle the mushrooms with a little of the rapeseed oil and season on both sides with salt and pepper. Cut the chorizo sausages in half lengthways.

2 Heat a large frying pan over a high heat and add the remaining oil. Lay in the chorizo, cut side down, along with the mushrooms, peeled side up, and cook for 3–4 minutes. Add 1 tablespoon of water to create a little steam before turning the chorizo and mushrooms over, adding the chopped garlic and frying for a further 4–5 minutes. If the mushrooms are really big, give them an extra few minutes and add a little more water. Just as they are cooked, add a squeeze of lemon juice and turn off the heat. Leave to rest.

3 Preheat the grill to its highest setting. Dress the watercress with the rest of the lemon juice, a little pepper and crumble in the feta cheese.

4 Cut the baps in half and toast them under the hot grill – I only toast the cut side. Remove the baps from the grill and press the toasted sides into the frying pan to soak up any juices that have run out of the mushrooms.

5 Place the mushroom on the bottom half of the bap along with the cooked chorizo sausage, and add a small handful of the watercress and feta salad. Put on the top half of the bap and enjoy.

ALMOND, RICOTTA AND CHERRY DROP SCONES

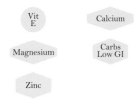

Vit E

Calcium

Magnesium

Carbs Low GI

Zinc

These make a great breakfast at the weekend, or you can make them in batches to freeze and eat whenever you like. The almonds make these scones rich in vitamin E, which is good for helping your skin stay supple and to prevent stretch marks. Ricotta is high in calcium – essential for baby's bones and teeth, which are now hardening. Calcium is also fantastic for combatting leg cramps and muscle spasms. The cherries add a really nice sweetness, as would dried cranberries or sultanas.

PREP TIME 10 MINUTES • COOK TIME 10 MINUTES • MAKES 12

50g dried cherries, chopped
zest and juice of 1 orange
50g ricotta cheese
2 tbsp runny honey
75ml almond milk or semi-
  skimmed cows' milk
1 free-range egg
1 tsp vanilla bean paste
  or extract
25g butter, melted
125g wholemeal or
  buckwheat flour
75g ground almonds
2 tbsp baking powder
pinch of salt
2–3 tbsp rapeseed oil

TO SERVE
2–3 tbsp ricotta cheese
2–3 tbsp flaked almonds
2 tbsp runny honey

1 Place the cherries and orange juice in a small bowl and microwave for 1 minute to plump up the cherries. Alternatively you can simmer the cherries and juice in a small saucepan for 5 minutes. Strain and discard the juice.

2 Combine the soaked cherries with the orange zest, ricotta, honey, milk, egg, vanilla and melted butter. Beat well until you form a loose mixture.

3 Mix the flour with the ground almonds, baking powder and salt in a large bowl. Make a well in the centre and pour in the wet mixture. Stir well to form a smooth paste.

4 Place a large frying pan over a medium heat and add some of the oil. Take 1 large tablespoon of the mixture and drop it into the hot frying pan. Repeat the process until you have formed 3 or 4 drop scones. Cook for 2–3 minutes, until bubbles start to rise in the wet mixture on top of the scones. Flip the scones over and cook for another 2–3 minutes. Remove the cooked scones to a plate. Adding a little more oil to the pan, repeat this process until you have used all the mixture.

5 Serve the warm drop scones with a little more ricotta, some flaked almonds and a drizzle of runny honey.

6 If you wish to freeze some of the drop scones, place a sheet of greaseproof paper in between each one and wrap well in cling film. Defrost before reheating in a pan, under the grill or in a warm oven.

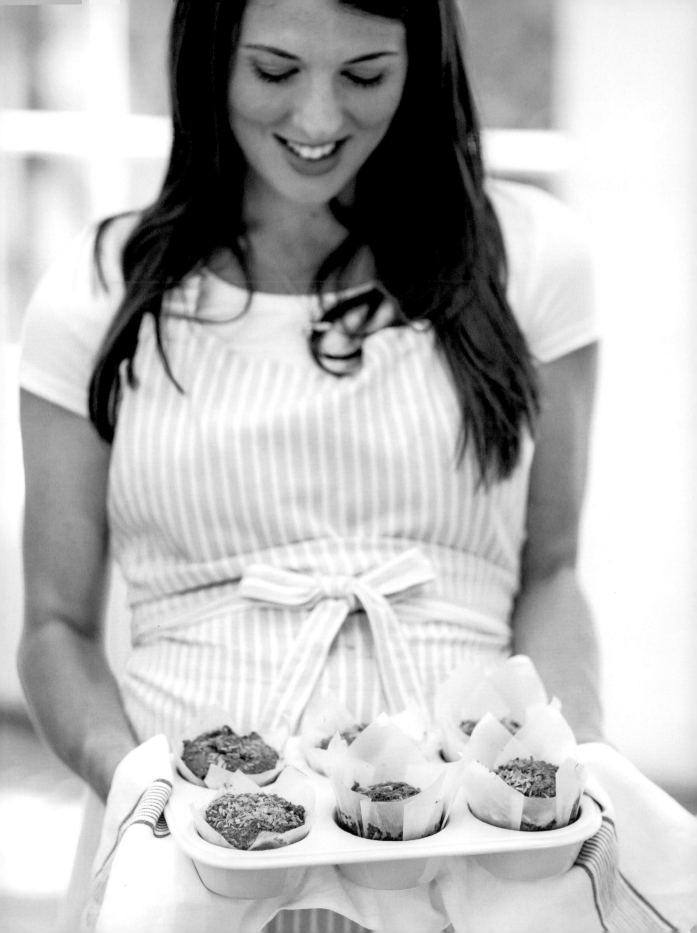

COCONUT AND BANANA MUFFINS

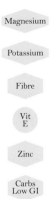

Magnesium

Potassium

Fibre

Vit
E

Zinc

Carbs
Low GI

These muffins are full of texture and flavour, and make a welcome change from the normal shop-bought variety. They are low in saturated fat, as they are made using coconut oil rather than butter, and high in fibre due to the addition of wheatbran. Despite being made without butter and sugar, these muffins are really lovely and moist, thanks to the coconut oil, with natural sweetness coming from the bananas and maple syrup.

The magnesium in the bran will help your baby to form the essential fatty acids and proteins it needs during these final and fast stages of development in the womb. Bananas offer a great source of energy for you, and also contain potassium, needed to help with vital muscle contraction during labour.

PREP TIME 15 MINUTES • COOK TIME 15–20 MINUTES • MAKES 12

125ml coconut oil, melted
100ml maple syrup
150ml coconut milk
3 ripe bananas, peeled and mashed
2 free-range eggs
150g wholemeal flour
125g wheatbran
2 tsp baking powder
2 tsp ground cinnamon
2 tbsp desiccated coconut, plus 2 tsp to sprinkle over before baking

1 Preheat the oven to 200°C (fan 180°C) and line a 12-hole muffin tray with muffin cases.

2 Mix all the wet ingredients together in a large bowl, including the mashed banana and the eggs. Whisk really well until everything is combined.

3 In a separate large bowl, mix the wholemeal flour with the wheatbran, baking powder, cinnamon and 2 tablespoons of desiccated coconut. Make a well in the centre and pour in half of the wet mixture. Mix well before adding the remaining wet mixture.

4 Spoon the batter into the muffin cases and sprinkle over the rest of the desiccated coconut. Bake in the oven for 20–25 minutes until the muffins are golden and well risen. Remove from the oven and leave to cool before eating.

5 Store these muffins in an airtight container to keep them fresh for up to 3 days. They are the perfect treat when you can't face a big brekkie.

BULGUR WHEAT, GOATS' CHEESE, GRAPE AND CELERY SALAD

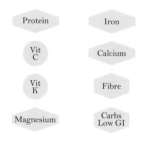

This is a naturally sweet and refreshing salad, full of raw fruits and vegetables, meaning extra fibre and nutrients for you and baby, as well as a little hit of fructose to satisfy a sweet tooth. I've added bulgur wheat for the iron and fibre content, but it will also help keep you feeling full. The goats' cheese, providing that it is pasteurised and not mould-ripened, is absolutely fine to eat and will add a welcome savoury note to this crunchy and sweet salad. You could also add a handful of watercress to up the iron and folate levels if you wish.

PREP TIME 10 MINUTES • COOK TIME 10 MINUTES • SERVES 2

50g bulgur wheat
2 apples, skin on and sliced
50g black grapes, halved
2 celery sticks, cut into 2cm pieces on the diagonal
50g pecans, chopped
75g soft goats' cheese, pasteurised and not mould-ripened
10 fresh mint leaves, finely chopped

FOR THE DRESSING
2 tsp Dijon mustard
2 tbsp cider vinegar
3 tbsp extra virgin rapeseed oil
1 tsp runny honey

1 Place a saucepan of water on the stove and bring to the boil. Once boiling, add the bulgur wheat and cook for 10 minutes until tender. Drain and leave to one side to cool slightly in the colander or sieve.

2 Make the dressing by adding all the ingredients to a small jar, placing on the lid and shaking hard for 30 seconds to combine everything together well.

3 Mix the apple, grapes, celery and chopped pecans in a bowl. Add the bulgur wheat and mix well. Crumble in the goats' cheese and mint, and season with plenty of salt and pepper. Pour over the dressing, give the salad a good stir and serve.

ASIAN SALMON LETTUCE CUPS

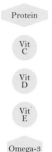

Protein

Vit
C

Vit
D

Vit
E

Omega-3

These salmon burgers are extremely tasty and can be rustled up in no time. Rather than serve them in a bun, which might be a bit heavy for dinner, I prefer to serve them in crunchy Chinese lettuce leaves – which are available in most large supermarkets and Asian supermarkets – along with dipping sauce and a crunchy raw slaw. If you can't find Chinese lettuce, iceberg is a good alternative. You can, of course, serve the salmon burgers in a bun if you fancy a more filling meal.

Salmon is one of the best sources of omega-3, which at this stage in your pregnancy is vital for baby's brain development.

PREP TIME 20 MINUTES • COOK TIME 20 MINUTES • SERVES 2

400g skinless and boneless salmon fillets
30g fresh coriander leaves
2cm piece fresh ginger, peeled and grated
2 garlic cloves, peeled and chopped
2 spring onions, trimmed and chopped
3 tbsp podded edamame beans (or defrosted peas)
2 tbsp rapeseed oil
salt and freshly ground black pepper

FOR THE SLAW
handful of bean sprouts
1 carrot, peeled and grated
10 fresh mint leaves
1 spring onion, trimmed and finely sliced
½ cucumber, peeled, deseeded and thinly sliced

FOR THE DIPPING SAUCE
6 tbsp rice wine vinegar
5cm piece fresh ginger, peeled and cut into fine strips
4 tsp agave nectar
2 tbsp sweet chilli sauce
juice of 1 lime

TO SERVE
4 Chinese lettuce leaves
2 lime wedges

1 Preheat the oven to 200°C (fan 180°C). Start by placing all the ingredients for the burger, except the rapeseed oil, in a food processor and blending until smooth. Season with salt and pepper and mould into 4 patties.

2 Heat the rapeseed oil in a frying pan over a medium heat and, when hot, lay in the salmon patties. The mixture may be a little wet but it will firm up as it cooks. Fry for 4–5 minutes on each side before transferring the fish cakes to a baking tray and cooking in the oven for a further 10 minutes.

3 While the burgers are cooking, make the slaw by combining all the prepared ingredients in a bowl.

4 Make the dipping sauce by combining all the ingredients in a small bowl and whisking them with a fork. Pour half of the sauce over the slaw.

5 Prepare the Chinese lettuce by separating the leaves and washing 4 of the biggest and juiciest-looking ones.

6 Now the salmon burgers should be ready. Remove the tray from the oven. Spoon some of the slaw into the Chinese lettuce leaves, and top each one with 1 of the burgers. Serve with a wedge of lime and a bowl of dipping sauce on the side. Roll the burgers tightly in the leaves to eat.

COURGETTE, MINT, PEA AND RICOTTA SALAD

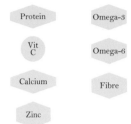

Protein

Vit C

Calcium

Zinc

Omega-3

Omega-6

Fibre

This is such a simple dish to make, and if, like me (currently 34 weeks pregnant and feeling rather large), you are in your third trimester of pregnancy at the height of summer, it will come as a welcome relief to have something that is easy to prepare, and light and easy to digest.

Everything in this salad is raw, which means that none of the nutrients will have been destroyed during cooking, thereby giving you optimum nutritional value. Flaxseed is an incredible source of omega-3, which is brain food for mum and baby, and will encourage your skin to stay supple, keeping stretch marks at bay. You can often develop stretch marks even after the baby is born, especially on your breasts, which will get larger if you are breastfeeding, so it's good to keep up your intake even in late pregnancy. Leave out the chilli if you're suffering from heartburn or indigestion.

PREP TIME 10 MINUTES • SERVES 2

4 courgettes, green and yellow if you can find them
3 handfuls of petits pois, defrosted
12 fresh mint leaves
zest and juice of 2 limes
2 tbsp avocado or flaxseed oil
2 tbsp pumpkin seeds
3 tbsp ricotta cheese
2 tbsp milled flaxseed
½ red chilli, deseeded and finely chopped (optional)
salt and freshly ground black pepper

1 Using a julienne speed peeler or just a normal speed peeler, slice the courgettes into ribbons and place in a large mixing bowl. If using a normal peeler, cut each ribbon into long, thin strips to make spaghetti. You can also use a spiralizer if you have one.

2 Put the petits pois in a bowl and squash gently using the back of a fork or your fingers. Add these to the courgettes. Shred the mint and mix with the peas and courgettes. Stir in the lime zest and juice, season with salt and pepper, and pour over the avocado or flaxseed oil. Add the pumpkin seeds and mix again.

3 Spoon the salad into serving bowls before adding the ricotta and garnishing with the milled flaxseed and chilli (if you are using it).

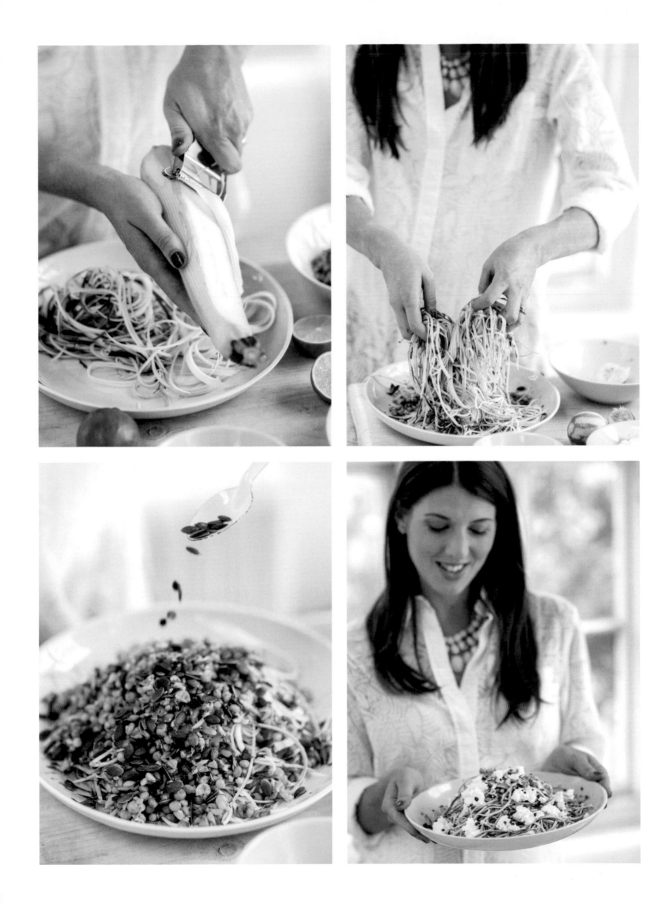

PRAWN AND ARTICHOKE WHOLEWHEAT SPAGHETTI

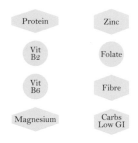

Protein | Zinc

Vit B2 | Folate

Vit B6 | Fibre

Magnesium | Carbs Low GI

I cooked this dish the other night when I was at home alone (currently 36 weeks pregnant) and fancied a little treat. It turned out so well that I simply had to include it here.

Artichokes are a good source of fibre and folate, both of which are extremely important in the final stages of your pregnancy. Folate works with vitamin B12, which is present in prawns, to produce red blood cells. B vitamins, also found in wholewheat pasta, have been associated with lower anxiety levels during pregnancy. Leave out the chilli if you're suffering from heartburn or indigestion.

PREP TIME 10 MINUTES • COOK TIME 15 MINUTES • SERVES 2

250g wholewheat spaghetti
2 tbsp rapeseed oil
3 spring onions, trimmed and finely sliced
1 garlic clove, peeled and finely chopped
1 tsp deseeded and finely chopped red chilli (optional)
12 cherry tomatoes, quartered
8 artichoke hearts in olive oil, drained and quartered
125g raw prawns
juice of 1 lemon
2 tbsp extra virgin olive oil
2 tbsp finely chopped flat-leaf parsley
salt and freshly ground black pepper

1 Start by cooking the spaghetti in a big saucepan of boiling salted water according to the packet instructions.

2 While the pasta is cooking, place a large frying pan over a medium heat and pour in the rapeseed oil. When hot, add in the spring onions, garlic, chilli (if using), tomatoes and the quartered artichokes, and fry for 3–4 minutes. Add the prawns and cook for a further 3–4 minutes, turning them over halfway through, until they are pink all over. Stir through the lemon juice and olive oil and turn off the heat.

3 Once the spaghetti is cooked, drain it well, reserving a little of the cooking liquid. Add this to the prawns, along with the cooked pasta and lots of black pepper and a large pinch of salt. Stir through the chopped parsley and serve piping hot.

PORK AND FENNEL FLATBREAD PIZZAS

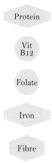

Protein

Vit B12

Folate

Iron

Fibre

This recipe is basically a cheat's pizza. It uses an unleavened bread dough for the base, so they are much quicker to make than regular pizzas. I am very lucky to have a butcher who makes amazing pork and fennel seed sausages, so I can skip the mixing stage of this recipe, and if you can get hold of some I recommend you do the same. Do make sure they contain fennel seeds, though, as these are great for indigestion. Pork is a good source of protein and vitamin B12, without which we can't absorb folate. Instead of the wholemeal flour, you can also make these with chickpea flour or another gluten-free alternative. Serve with a simple rocket salad dressed with a squeeze of lemon juice and some olive oil.

PREP TIME 40 MINUTES • COOK TIME 20 MINUTES • SERVES 2

FOR THE FLATBREAD
260g wholemeal flour
150ml natural yogurt
50ml milk of your choosing
2 tsp baking powder
½ tsp fennel seeds, crushed
1 tsp salt
2 tbsp rapeseed oil

FOR THE MEATBALLS
4 pork and fennel sausages,
    or 300g minced pork,
    1 tsp fennel seeds,
    crushed, 2 tbsp finely
    chopped flat-leaf parsley
    and salt and freshly
    ground black pepper

FOR THE TOPPING
100g cooked spinach
    (or defrosted frozen)
150g mascarpone cheese
1 garlic clove, peeled
    and grated
zest and juice of 1 lemon
extra virgin olive oil
salt and freshly ground
    black pepper

TO SERVE
4 tbsp extra virgin olive oil
15g Parmesan cheese,
    shaved

1 Preheat the oven to 210°C (fan 190°C). Make the flatbreads by combining the flour with the yogurt, milk, baking powder, fennel seeds and the salt in a large bowl. Mix to form a dough then knead lightly until smooth – no longer than a minute or so. Split the dough into 4 small balls and roll out on a floured surface to a thickness of about 2mm.

2 Heat a large griddle pan or frying pan over a high heat. One at a time, drizzle a little of the rapeseed oil over each side of a flatbread and place in the hot pan. Cook for 2–3 minutes on each side. It should be slightly golden brown. Lay the cooked flatbread on a baking tray and repeat the process until you have cooked all of them.

3 Now make the meatballs. If using sausages, remove the meat from their skins and mould into 20 mini-meatballs. If you are making it yourself, mix the minced pork with the fennel seeds, parsley and seasoning, and mould into 20 small balls.

4 For the topping, blend the cooked spinach with 100g of the mascarpone cheese, the garlic, lemon juice and zest, and season well with salt and pepper. This mixture doesn't need to be smooth and can be done by hand or in a blender.

5 Spread the spinach and mascarpone mixture over the base of each flatbread. Place 5 meatballs on each and spoon on the remaining mascarpone. Drizzle generously with extra virgin olive oil and cook in the oven for 15 minutes. Remove from the oven and top with the shaved Parmesan and more olive oil.

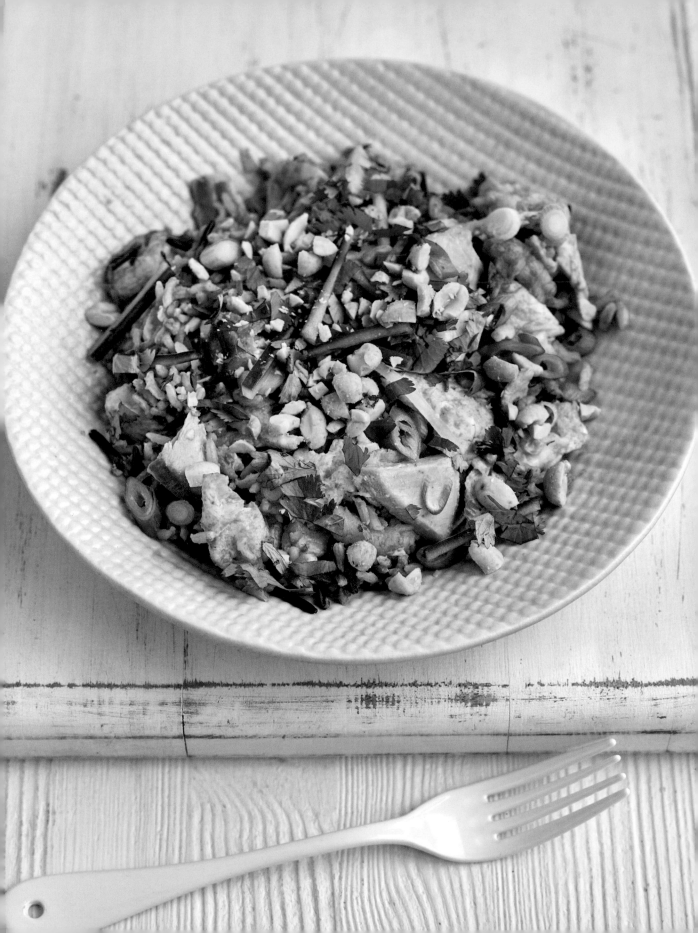

INDONESIAN RICE POT WITH EGG AND SALMON (NASI GORENG)

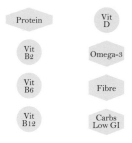

Protein

Vit
D

Vit
B2

Omega-3

Vit
B6

Fibre

Vit
B12

Carbs
Low GI

This is traditionally made with white rice, as most Asian dishes containing rice tend to be, but with health always at the forefront of my mind I've substituted brown rice mixed with a little wild rice for extra fibre and added B vitamins. Eggs and salmon both contain vitamin D, something most of us should get in sufficient amounts from the sun; however, if you are pregnant in the winter it's really important that you eat a fair amount as well, especially during the third trimester. Lack of vitamin D can lead to your baby having weak bones. Leave out the chilli if you're suffering from heartburn or indigestion.

PREP TIME 15 MINUTES • COOK TIME 35 MINUTES • SERVES 2

300g brown rice
50g wild rice
2½ tbsp rapeseed oil,
    plus extra for greasing
200g skinless salmon fillet
3 free-range eggs, beaten
6 spring onions, trimmed
    and sliced
2 garlic cloves, peeled
    and finely chopped
5cm piece fresh ginger,
    peeled and finely
    chopped
2 tsp ground turmeric
2 tbsp tomato purée
75g small prawns
2 tbsp soy sauce
1 tbsp fish sauce
juice of 2 limes
salt

TO SERVE
½ cucumber, deseeded
    and cut into matchsticks
2 spring onions, trimmed
    and thinly sliced
1 red chilli, deseeded
    and sliced (optional)
1 tbsp plain peanuts,
    toasted and chopped
handful of fresh coriander
    leaves, chopped

1 Cook the brown rice and wild rice according to packet instructions, until tender – use separate pans if they require different lengths of time. Once cooked, drain the rice and leave to cool.

2 Preheat the grill to its highest setting and lightly oil a baking tray. Lay the salmon on the tray and brush it all over with half a tablespoon of the oil and sprinkle over a little salt. Cook under the hot grill for 8 minutes before turning off the heat and allowing the residual heat to cook it through. You can also steam the salmon if you prefer.

3 Pour 1 tablespoon of the oil into a wok or sauté pan and turn the heat up high. Add the beaten eggs to the hot oil and scramble them until they are firm; this will take around 2–3 minutes. Remove the eggs to a plate and leave to one side.

4 Add the remaining oil to the wok and add the spring onions, garlic and ginger. Fry for 2–3 minutes before stirring in the turmeric and tomato purée and cook for 2 minutes. Now add the cooked rice and prawns, and flake in the cooked salmon and egg. Stir in the soy sauce, fish sauce and lime juice, and heat through over a medium heat for 3–4 minutes.

5 Spoon into serving bowls and garnish with the cucumber, spring onions, chilli (if using) and peanuts. Add a scattering of coriander and serve.

COURGETTE, PANCETTA AND KALE CARBONARA

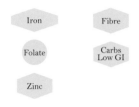

Iron

Folate

Zinc

Fibre

Carbs
Low GI

I love this dinner! It's quick, simple and tastes amazing. It's so important to add greens to your diet when you can, and I find that adding them to dishes like pasta, tray bakes and casseroles is so much more interesting than just having them steamed on the side.

The zinc in the wholewheat pasta will continue to help baby's brain develop to its full potential while in the womb, and the fibre will help keep your digestive system working nicely, which is important to keep energy levels up during the final stages of pregnancy.

PREP TIME 10 MINUTES • COOK TIME 15–20 MINUTES • SERVES 2

250g wholewheat
   penne pasta
1 tbsp rapeseed oil
125g smoked pancetta
2 garlic cloves, peeled and
   grated or finely chopped
100g kale
3 courgettes, green and
   yellow if you can find
   them, trimmed
   and grated
4 heaped tbsp crème fraîche
zest and juice of 1 lemon
25g walnuts, chopped
50g Parmesan cheese,
   grated
10 fresh basil leaves
salt and freshly ground
   black pepper

1 Start by cooking your pasta in a big saucepan of boiling salted water according to the packet instructions. While the pasta is cooking, you can start to make the sauce.

2 Place a large frying pan over a high heat and add the oil. When hot, add the pancetta and fry for 3–4 minutes, until it is slightly golden brown. Now add the garlic, cook for another minute and then turn off the heat. Leave the pan on the stove.

3 When the pasta is 2 minutes away from being cooked, add the kale into the boiling water with the pasta. Once the pasta is cooked and the kale is just wilted, drain both, keeping back 2–3 tablespoons of the cooking liquid, and add the pasta and kale to the cooked pancetta. Season with lots of black pepper and a little salt. Place the pan back over a medium heat and mix in the grated courgettes, crème fraîche, and lemon zest and juice.

4 Stir the pasta, letting it heat through for a few minutes, wilting the courgettes, then serve. Sprinkle with the chopped walnuts and grated Parmesan, and tear over the basil leaves.

MAPLE AND THYME ROASTED CHICKEN WITH PARSNIP CHIPS

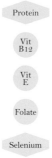

Protein

Vit B12

Vit E

Folate

Selenium

Nothing beats the flavours of a roast dinner, but unfortunately roast dinners can be a bit of a faff to make, especially if you are heavily pregnant! I cook this chicken with parsnips quite regularly, as it takes hardly any time at all to prepare, the ingredients are easily accessible and it's good for you.

Chicken, especially the free-range variety, is a really good source of selenium, which baby needs now more than ever as it is partly responsible for laying down good fat supplies and for the ongoing production of skin and hair. Hazelnuts are a rich source of vitamin E, very important if you're trying to prevent stretch marks.

PREP TIME 15 MINUTES • COOK TIME 40 MINUTES • SERVES 2

1 x 800g–1kg free-range chicken or 2 x 300g chicken legs
3 tbsp rapeseed oil
3 tbsp maple syrup
4 parsnips, peeled and cut into wedges
200g Chantenay carrots, washed
2 fresh thyme sprigs, leaves picked
salt and freshly ground black pepper

FOR THE DRESSING
100g roasted hazelnuts
25g flat-leaf parsley
zest and juice of 1 lemon
2 tsp Dijon mustard
4 tbsp extra virgin rapeseed oil
1 tsp red wine vinegar
salt and freshly ground black pepper

1 Preheat the oven to 200°C (fan 180°C). Prepare the chicken by turning it on to its breast, revealing the backbone. Using a pair of sharp kitchen scissors, cut down either side of the back bone from the bottom end to the neck. Once you have cut both sides, you should be able to remove the backbone quite easily. Discard this or save it for stock (page 155). You now have a spatchcocked chicken, which you need to cut in two. Take a large sharp knife and cut straight through the breastbone, leaving you with 2 halves, each with one with a leg and a breast.

2 Rub each half of the chicken, or the chicken legs, if using, with 1 tablespoon each of rapeseed oil and maple syrup, and season with salt and pepper. Lay on a large baking tray and cook in the oven for 10 minutes.

3 Remove the tray from the oven and scatter the parsnips and carrots around the chicken. Sprinkle with the thyme leaves, drizzle the vegetables with the remaining oil and maple syrup, and season with a little salt and some black pepper. Roast for a further 30 minutes.

4 While the chicken is cooking you can make the dressing. In a small blender, blitz all the ingredients to form a chunky paste. Alternatively, you can chop the dry ingredients by hand or grind them in a pestle and mortar, then mix in the wet ingredients and taste for seasoning.

5 Remove the now caramelised and cooked chicken, parsnips and carrots from the oven and serve with the hazelnut dressing.

THE ULTIMATE CHICKEN AND AVOCADO BURGER

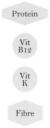

Protein

Vit
B12

Vit
K

Fibre

When I asked pregnant women what they most wanted to eat during pregnancy, I usually got the same answer: A BURGER! In particular from my amazing neighbour Vicki, who is supermum to two delicious twin boys and practically lived on burgers for her entire pregnancy! I'm sitting here now, 37 weeks pregnant, and honestly, it's all I can think about. They are packed with protein and iron and are the ultimate comfort food, and so I just had to include a recipe for one, but of course with a healthy spin. Vicki, this one is for you.

PREP TIME 20 MINUTES • COOK TIME 15 MINUTES • SERVES 2

2 x 200g skinless free-range
    chicken breasts
2 tbsp rapeseed oil
juice of 1 lemon
1 ripe avocado
2 wholemeal burger buns
2 heaped tsp mayonnaise
    (made with
    pasteurised egg)
2 tsp Dijon mustard
1 plum tomato, thinly sliced
1 large pickled gherkin,
    thinly sliced
1 baby gem lettuce, leaves
    separated and washed
salt and freshly ground
    black pepper

TO SERVE
Sweet Potato Chips
    (see page 82)

1 First, butterfly the chicken breasts. Place one hand on top of the breast and use a sharp knife to cut most of the way through the breast from top to bottom, and then open it up as you would a book. This will make your chicken cook more evenly. Drizzle the chicken with 1 tablespoon of the rapeseed oil and half of the the lemon juice, and season with salt and pepper.

2 Heat a griddle or frying pan over a medium heat. Cook the seasoned chicken breasts on the hot griddle for 8 minutes on each side. They should be well browned, with char marks from the griddle pan. You can also cook the chicken breasts under a hot grill for the same amount of time.

3 While the chicken is cooking, cut the avocado in half, remove the stone and scoop out the flesh using a spoon. Cut the flesh into small chunks and place in a bowl. Use a fork to mash the avocado slightly. Season with a little salt and pepper and the remaining rapeseed oil and lemon juice. Mix well.

4 Once cooked, remove the chicken from the griddle or grill and leave it to rest on a plate, covered with foil.

5 Toast the cut sides of the burger buns either under the grill or on the griddle until slightly golden and crispy.

6 Smother the bottom half of each bun with mayonnaise and the top half with Dijon mustard. Place the cooked chicken breast on the bottom, followed by a large serving of avocado. Top with slices of tomato, gherkin and lettuce, and put on the top half of the bun. Squish it down a little to prevent your artwork falling over and enjoy with some sweet potato chips.

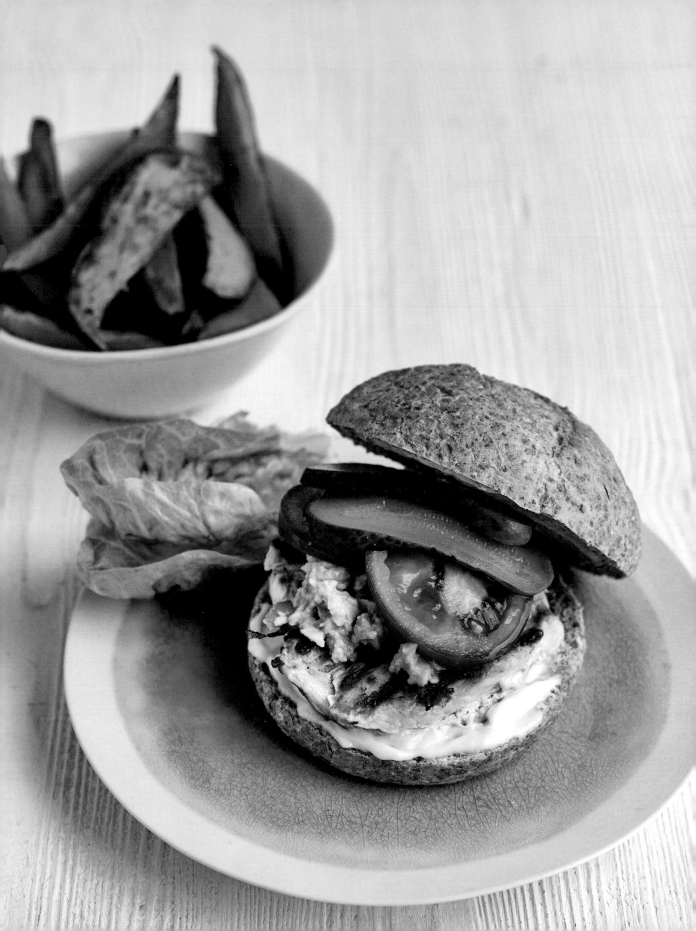

POACHED TURKEY, MANGO, ALFALFA AND CASHEW NUT SALAD

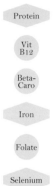

Protein

Vit B12

Beta-Caro

Iron

Folate

Selenium

I really enjoy inventing new salads and making them taste truly delicious. I like thinking about the colours, textures and different ingredients I can incorporate to create something that will make my taste buds sing. This salad is Asian-inspired, using fruit – in this case mango – to add sweetness, which works really well with the tender and super-healthy turkey. Mangos are a rich source of beta-carotene, which will help support your baby's immune system. Cashews are rich in iron, needed to keep anaemia and fatigue at bay, and I've added alfalfa sprouts, which are lovely and rich in folate. At this stage, in the third trimester, folate will help to get your baby's immune system working, which will help to fight off infection when your baby is born.

PREP TIME 15 MINUTES • COOK TIME 15 MINUTES • SERVES 2

300g skinless free-range turkey or chicken breast
4 tbsp cashew nuts
1 large ripe mango
½ cucumber, cut in half lengthways, deseeded and cut into fine strips
2 spring onions, trimmed and cut into fine strips
2 handfuls of bean sprouts
50g alfalfa sprouts

FOR THE DRESSING
juice of 2 limes
1 tsp sesame oil
3 tbsp light soy sauce
1 tsp agave nectar

TO SERVE
1 tbsp sesame seeds
6–8 fresh mint leaves

1 First poach the turkey. Bring a saucepan of water or chicken stock to the boil. Turn the heat down to a simmer and add the turkey breast. Cook for about 15 minutes or until the turkey is cooked through. Remove from the hot broth and leave to cool on a plate while you prepare the rest of the salad.

2 Make the dressing by combining all the ingredients in a small bowl. Leave to one side.

3 Toast the cashew nuts in a dry frying pan set over a high heat for 2–3 minutes, shaking the pan often, until they are slightly golden brown. Turn off the heat and transfer the cashews to a small bowl.

4 Slice the mango down either side of the flat stone which runs through the middle. Cut each cheek into 4 wedges and cut the flesh away from the skin in the same way you would a melon. Cut the peeled mango into bite-sized pieces or thin strips.

5 Mix the mango with the cucumber and spring onions. Add the bean sprouts and alfalfa sprouts and stir through the toasted cashew nuts.

6 When the turkey is cool enough to handle, shred it into fine pieces and add to the salad. Mix well before pouring over all of the dressing. Serve with a sprinkling of sesame seeds and a scattering of fresh mint.

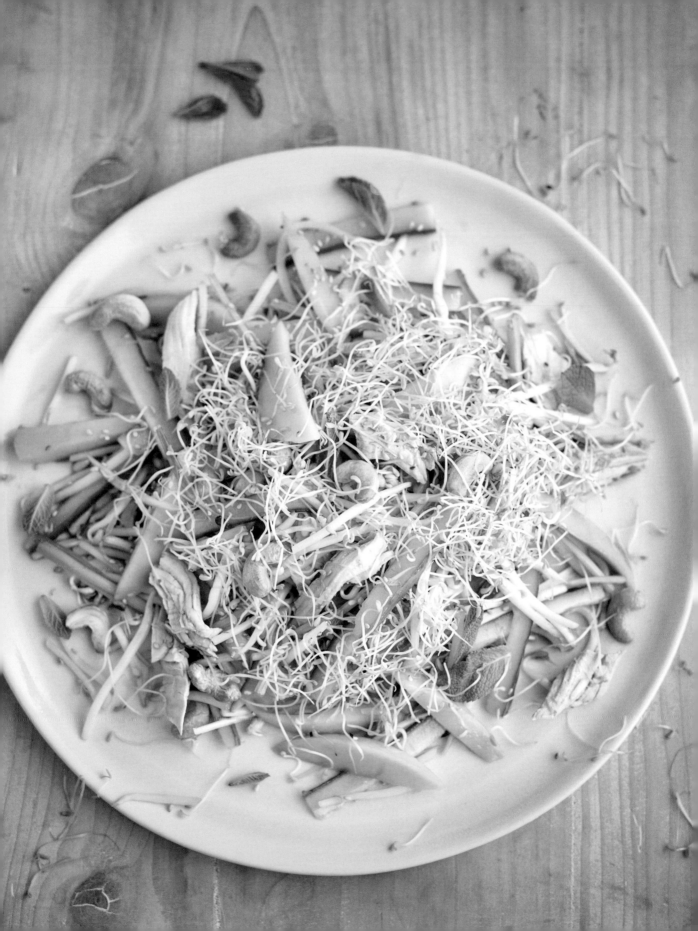

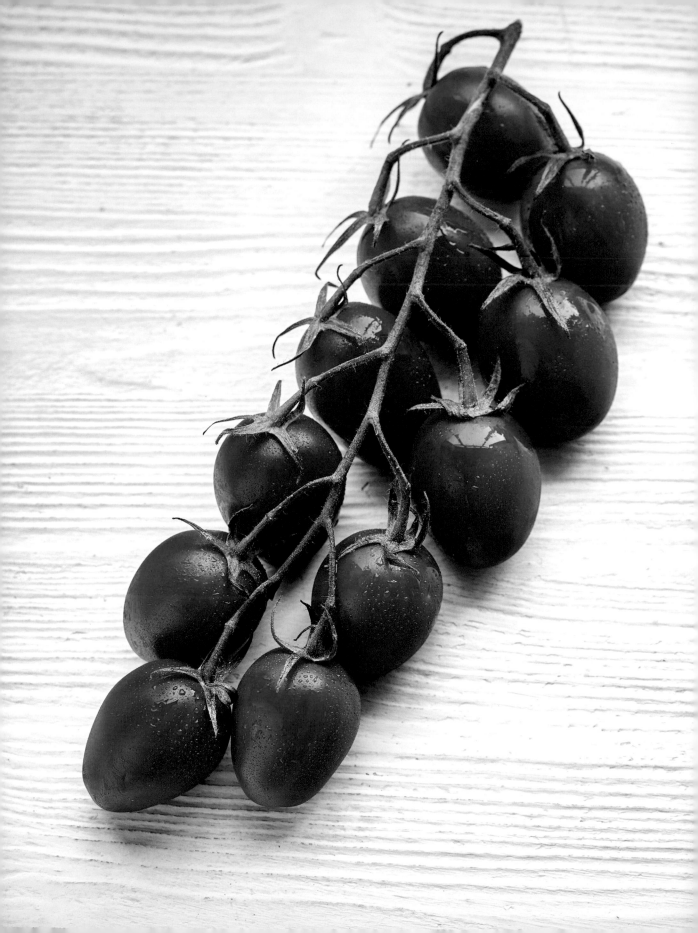

NESTING

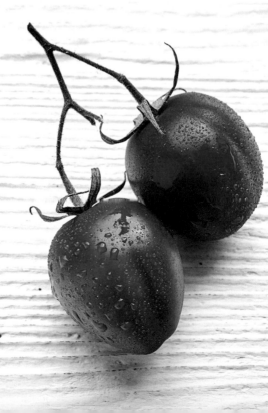

When I started thinking about the chapters that were going to make up this book, this was one of the most obvious. Of course I needed to make sure I included recipes to see you through your pregnancy, but I also needed to think about what you were going to eat once your little one came along. As I speak to more and more mums, one of the things that comes up time and again is how much your life is turned upside down for the first six weeks (or perhaps six years!) after having your baby. Your life is no longer your own and the thought of cooking an evening meal is sometimes going to be a daunting one, let alone shopping for it, especially in the beginning.

I know that many mums approaching their due date will take time off before baby is born to make the house and baby's room look perfect, ensuring all clothes are ironed and hospital bags packed, but I think that the idea of stocking up your freezer with good home-cooked meals is also a necessity. I'm not suggesting that you do all the cooking – perhaps someone else can make a dish or two and, of course, I'm sure your partner is capable of spending a couple of hours in the kitchen one Sunday afternoon preparing a few batches of Classic Beef Ragù (page 140). If you make some of the dishes from this chapter and have them stashed in the freezer, at least you know you'll have something to fall back on in the first few weeks of being a new mum.

Ready meals and convenience food are OK every now and then, but remember that your body will have just been through the amazing yet challenging experience of giving birth, and you will still be in recovery mode. Add to this lack of sleep and the responsibility of caring for a new person, and you could run the risk of becoming run down. A healthy diet, consisting of home-cooked food, is nature's best healer and will give you the much-needed energy required to get you through the first tough weeks.

You may or may not be breastfeeding, but if you are, your body is just as responsible as it was when you were pregnant for providing all the nutrients and minerals that your baby needs on a daily basis to grow big and strong, and fight off infection and improve his or her immune system. Breastfeeding can really take its toll on your energy levels, and it's vital you keep up your calorie intake with healthy and nutritious food, and don't overload on instant energy and empty calories. The NHS recommends that, while breastfeeding, you consume an extra 500 calories per day. Processed food, although convenient, will not provide any goodness for you or baby, leaving you both undernourished and tired.

The recipes in this chapter are all healthy and wholesome, but also freezer-friendly, so therefore won't contain all the fresh fruits and vegetables that you need on a daily basis. You still need to add some steamed greens or vegetables to your meals, and perhaps a jacket potato or some boiled wholegrain rice, but these dishes this will provide the main bulk of what you need.

I have tried to make sure these recipes are 'fork-feeding friendly' too. This idea came from my Auntie Julie, who has had three children. She said that the second you sit down to eat a meal, the baby will inevitably start to cry and need a cuddle or a feed. So the majority of these recipes can be eaten using a fork only, leaving you with one hand free to tend to baby as you eat your rather rushed and probably cold, but perfectly nourishing and wholesome, home-cooked meal.

This chapter is intended to make your life easier, and will hopefully give you some new recipes to add to your family's repertoire once life starts getting back to some form of normality. It includes some of my favourite family recipes, and I'm so happy to be able to share them with you.

What to expect after the birth

POST DELIVERY: After giving birth, regardless of how your delivery went, you will be exhausted. Your body has been through a challenge and whether you had a natural delivery lasting two hours or many more hours, or a C-section, you are going to be feeling extremely weak and like you have just run three marathons, one after the other, in stilettos! No wonder it's us girls that got tasked with the job of carrying and delivering babies... You will need plenty of rest and a good diet to help you get back to your old self. You will also need to keep up your iron levels because you will have lost some blood during delivery – you can find this in lots of leafy green vegetables and, of course, in red meat. Pulses are also great.

BREASTFEEDING: If you choose to breastfeed, then the baby is going to be draining you of essential nutrients and vitamins as you are still going to be nourishing your little one as you did when he or she was inside you. Calcium is very important as breastfeeding without sufficient supplies of calcium can lead to brittle bones when you are older. A glass of milk, a small lump of cheese or a yogurt or two a day will help provide sufficient amounts. It's also important to remember to drink plenty of water as this will help your milk production and it can also help prevent milks ducts from blocking, which can lead to developing very painful and unpleasant mastitis. Fenugreek seeds have also been shown to be very good for milk production; try them crushed into a glass of water or in a cup of hot tea. Omega-3 and essential fatty acids are needed for good brain development in your baby as it progresses and grows. These can be found in oily fish such as salmon, mackerel, sardines and trout.

WEIGHT LOSS: You can expect to lose around 4–8 kilos during the first week or so after delivery. Around 2–4 kilos from the baby, up to 1 kilo from the placenta and 1–3 kilos in water. It's important to keep hydrated during this time. Don't rush trying to lose any additional 'baby weight' though – the next few weeks and months are all about looking after you and baby, so don't hurry to get back into your skinny jeans! There is plenty of time for that later. Just enjoy the wonderful journey your body has been through and marvel at how amazing women's bodies are.

DIGESTION: Your digestion will likely be a bit out of sorts after the delivery and it may be a few days before you can actually 'properly' go to the loo. This is completely normal. Many women are nervous about going to the loo, especially after a natural delivery: don't be. Drinking plenty of water will help to speed things up. Eat plenty of fresh fruit, vegetables and wholegrains for fibre, and perhaps add in a few prunes or a little Earl Grey and Ginger Prune Compote from page 95 and wait for nature's call!

SLEEPLESS NIGHTS: Although you love your baby unconditionally, oh, how you wish he or she would sleep! Until your baby has settled into a bit more of a routine, all you can do is take care of yourself and sleep whenever you can, especially in the first few weeks when your body is still recovering from the labour. A good, nutritious and protein-rich diet full of meat, eggs, fish and pulses will help with energy levels. Drink plenty of water and allow yourself a few snacks for boosts of energy (see the Healthy Snacks and Sweet Treats chapters, pages 168–203). Don't forget you are advised to eat up to 500 extra calories per day if breastfeeding, so make the most of it and do all you can to get through the tough first few months. Keep going Mum – you are doing so amazingly well!

BABY BLUES: Giving birth is a huge life-changing event. Combined with a huge surge in your hormone levels about five days afterwards, and the fact that you will probably be feeling totally overwhelmed by the amazing but surreal experience of having a baby to care for while not getting enough sleep, and it's no wonder many women report feeling like they're on an emotional roller coaster. Potassium and magnesium are great for helping lift your mood, acting as nature's tranquilliser. Seeds, nuts, dried fruits, leafy green vegetables and wholegrains contain these in abundance. Folate, present in leafy greens, and zinc, present in most meat and dairy and pulses will also help. The vitamin B family, especially vitamin B12, found in lean meat, eggs, fish, dairy and soya, is also good for boosting your mood. For most women, the baby blues will pass quite quickly and you will soon be laughing about the fact that you cried about not being able to decide which top to wear that day, or the fact that you couldn't find anything you fancied eating in the fridge. However, if you do find that you are still feeling down 4–6 weeks after the birth of your baby, speak to your GP or health visitor. They will be able to give you advice and assist in more serious cases of possible postnatal depression, which is very common and highly treatable. You are not alone and there is lots of help available.

CLASSIC BEEF RAGÙ

Protein

Vit B12

Zinc

A classic beef ragù is something we should all have in our repertoire, and this is my go-to recipe that I have used for ever. I use this to make everything from lasagne (or my twist on it, Ravioli Lasagne, see opposite) to spaghetti bolognese, cannelloni or even cottage pie. It's so reassuring to know you have a batch or two in the freezer that can be defrosted easily, leaving you with an effortless yet tasty and nutritious meal when time is precious. Beef ragù is high in protein and iron, which will help fight fatigue and boost energy levels – essential during those sleepless nights!

PREP TIME 10 MINUTES • COOK TIME 45 MINUTES • MAKES 4 PORTIONS

2 tbsp rapeseed oil
1 large carrot, peeled and finely chopped
2 celery sticks, finely chopped
1 large red onion, peeled and finely chopped
100g pancetta
500g minced beef, lean and organic, if possible
3 garlic cloves, peeled and finely chopped
2 tsp dried oregano
1 tbsp flour
3 large tbsp tomato purée
250ml red wine
500ml hot beef stock
2 bay leaves
salt and freshly ground black pepper

1 Heat the oil in a large casserole pan over a medium heat. When hot, add the carrot, celery and red onion. Cover with the lid and cook for 5–6 minutes to soften the vegetables, stirring once or twice to ensure nothing burns. Increase the heat and add the pancetta. Cook for a few minutes, until the pancetta is slightly golden and its fat has melted.

2 Add the minced beef, garlic and dried oregano. Stir to coat the mince in all the juices and allow the meat to brown completely; this will take about 3 minutes. Now add the flour and tomato purée, mix well to coat the meat and cook for 2–3 minutes.

3 Pour in the red wine and bring the mixture to the boil so that the alcohol boils off. After 2–3 minutes, add the hot stock. Season well with salt and pepper, add the bay leaves and leave to simmer for between 45 minutes and 1 hour. The ragù is now ready to use or you can freeze it in portion sizes that work for your family. Make sure you label the freezer bags with the date you made it. The ragù will keep in the freezer for up to 1 month.

4 When you want to eat the ragù, defrost it fully in the fridge overnight before reheating it in a saucepan or in the microwave until piping hot. If using a microwave, place in a microwavable bowl, cover with a plate or cling film and cook for 3–4 minutes, then stir and heat for a further 3–4 minutes until piping hot all the way through. Times may vary depending on the strength of your microwave. If using a saucepan, empty the contents of the bag into a medium-sized pan. Add 3–4 tablespoons of water and heat until it starts to boil, then simmer for 5 minutes.

RAVIOLI LASAGNE

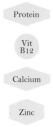

Protein

Vit
B12

Calcium

Zinc

This is the sort of food I crave when I feel like I need a big hug, and I've been assured that for the first few weeks after the birth, that is exactly how I am going to feel. It's rich in protein and the pasta's slow-releasing energy will see you through the long night feeds. I use shop-bought fresh ravioli or tortellini for this dish. It's so much easier to mix everything together and top with cheese sauce than layering in the traditional way, and is something a little different to look forward to after a day spent tending to babe. Serve with a simple rocket salad or some peppery watercress for a rich iron hit.

PREP TIME 15 MINUTES • COOK TIME 45 MINUTES • MAKES 4 PORTIONS

400g good quality fresh
    ravioli (I usually go
    for ones stuffed with
    spinach and ricotta)
200g fresh baby leaf spinach
1 x portion of Classic Beef
    Ragù (see opposite)

FOR THE CHEESE
    SAUCE
30g butter
30g plain flour
1 pint cows' milk
80g Cheddar
    cheese, grated
20g Parmesan
    cheese, grated
1 tbsp Dijon mustard
1 large pinch of
    grated nutmeg
salt and freshly ground
    black pepper

1 Preheat the oven to 210°C (fan 190°C) if you plan to eat the lasagne straight away. To make the cheese sauce, melt the butter in a small saucepan, then add all the flour and stir well to make a paste. Cook for a few minutes then pour in half the milk. Whisk well to remove any lumps and bring to the boil. When you have a smooth, very thick sauce, add the rest of the milk and repeat the process, then simmer for 5 minutes to cook out the flour. Add the cheeses and mustard, and season with plenty of pepper, a little salt and pinch of nutmeg.

2 Gently reheat the ragù until piping hot. If using a microwave, place in a microwavable bowl, cover with a plate or some cling film and cook for 3–4 minutes, stir and heat for a further 3–4 minutes. Times may vary depending on the strength of your microwave. If using in a saucepan, empty the contents of the bag into a medium-sized pan. Add 3–4 tablespons of water and heat until it starts to boil, then simmer for 5 minutes.

3 Boil the ravioli for 30 seconds in a large pan of salted water. Drain, retaining 3–4 tablespoons of the water. Return the pasta to the pan, along with the cooking water, and mix in the ragù over a very low heat. Fold in the spinach, stirring until it wilts.

4 Pour the ravioli and ragù into 1 large or 2 small baking dishes (either disposable for ease of freezing and storing, or ceramic if eating now). Pour over the cheese sauce and finish with a little grated Parmesan. If you are eating the lasagne today, cook in the oven for 30–45 minutes until browned and bubbling. If freezing, cool completely then cover with cling film, label with the date and freeze for up to 1 month. Defrost fully overnight in the fridge before cooking in a 190°C (fan 170°C) oven for 30–45 minutes until piping hot.

BEEF MASSAMAN

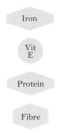

Iron

Vit E

Protein

Fibre

This curry is not hot at all, making it great for breastfeeding mums. The spices I use are gentle and warming and will help keep your immune system in full working order. The beef is naturally very high in iron, which is really important when breastfeeding, and the coconut milk is a great source of vitamin E, essential for helping your skin recover from all the stretching during pregnancy. If you have a slow cooker, this is the perfect dish to prepare in it, as the beef needs plenty of time to become tender and to absorb all the delicious aromatics; simply cook all the ingredients together in the slow cooker for 8 hours on a low setting.

PREP TIME 20 MINUTES • COOK TIME 2½ HOURS • MAKES 6 PORTIONS

800g beef shin, cut into roughly 5cm pieces
2 tbsp rapeseed oil
400ml coconut milk
juice of 3 limes
1 tsp agave syrup
500g potatoes, peeled and cut into 5cm chunks
salt
fresh coriander leaves, to serve

FOR THE CURRY PASTE
2 dried large red chillies, split in half
2 tbsp coriander seeds
2 tbsp cumin seeds
4 cloves
2 cinnamon sticks, halved
6 peppercorns
10cm piece ginger, peeled and roughly chopped
2 sticks of lemon grass, roughly chopped
4 garlic cloves, peeled
30g fresh coriander
1 tbsp fish sauce
1 tsp shrimp paste
2 tbsp tomato purée

1 First make the curry paste. Toast the chillies, coriander and cumin seeds, cloves, cinnamon and peppercorns in a dry frying pan set over a medium heat for 2–3 minutes, shaking the pan often, until fragrant. Transfer to a pestle and mortar (or a spice grinder or mini food processor) and grind to a fine paste. Add the rest of the ingredients for the paste, and grind until smooth. Coat the beef pieces well in the curry paste.

2 Heat the oil in a large wok over a high heat. Add the coated beef and season with salt. Cook for 4–5 minutes, until browned on all sides, then pour in the coconut milk, the juice of 1 lime and the agave syrup. Reduce the heat, cover and simmer for 2 hours.

3 Stir through the potatoes and cook for a further 40 minutes. Keep an eye on the curry and if it looks as though it is starting to dry out, add a little water. Once the meat is very tender and the potatoes are cooked, the curry is ready. Add the remaining lime juice. Taste to ensure the flavours are well balanced: the curry should be sweet, sour, salty and a little hot without being spicy. You may need a squeeze more lime or an extra dash of fish sauce.

4 Either eat straight away or cool before portioning into labelled freezer bags. Freeze for up to 1 month. Ensure to defrost it fully overnight in the fridge before reheating. If using a microwave, place in a microwavable bowl, cover with a plate or cling film and cook for 3–4 minutes. Stir and heat for a further 3–4 minutes until piping hot all the way through. Times may vary depending on the strength of your microwave. If using a saucepan, empty the contents into a medium-sized pan. Add 3–4 tablespoons of water, bring to the boil, then simmer for 5 minutes. Sprinkle with fresh coriander before serving.

LAMB, SULTANA AND PINE-NUT MEATBALLS

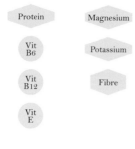

Protein

Vit B6

Vit B12

Vit E

Magnesium

Potassium

Fibre

Lamb and dried fruit have a natural affinity and this dish reminds me of the Middle Eastern cuisine that I love so much. Lamb is a good source of protein, needed for energy and general recovery after the birth. Vitamin B12, also present in lamb, is essential for proper functioning of the nervous system and the formation of red blood cells. Vitamin B12 is passed to your baby in breast milk, so it is important to keep up sufficient supplies if you are breastfeeding. I make a little tomato sauce to coat the meatballs in so they stay nice and moist as they freeze. Then all I need to do is cook some brown rice or soak couscous in stock and serve them with Greek yogurt on the side. They also go brilliantly with the Bulgur Wheat Salad on page 61.

PREP TIME 20 MINUTES • COOK TIME 30 MINUTES • MAKES 4 PORTIONS

FOR THE MEATBALLS
600g minced lamb
75g sultanas, roughly chopped
75g pine nuts, toasted and chopped
15g flat-leaf parsley, finely chopped
1 free-range egg yolk
1 tsp ground cumin
pinch of ground cinnamon
small pinch of dried chilli flakes
2 tbsp rapeseed oil
salt and freshly ground black pepper

FOR THE SAUCE
2 tbsp rapeseed oil
1 large red onion, peeled and finely chopped
2 garlic cloves, peeled and finely chopped
1 tsp ground cumin
small pinch of dried chilli flakes
½ tsp brown sugar
500ml tomato passata
300ml chicken stock
salt and freshly ground black pepper

1 Start by making the sauce. Heat the oil in a saucepan over a medium heat. Add the onion and sweat for 3–4 minutes, stirring occasionally, before adding the garlic, cumin and chilli flakes. Season with salt and pepper and add the sugar. Pour in the passata and stock, then let it simmer over a low heat for 15 minutes while you make the meatballs.

2 Place all the ingredients except for the oil in a large bowl and season with salt and pepper. Mix together well, but don't overwork the mixture. Then, using the palms of your hands, shape into 16 balls.

3 Heat the oil in a frying pan over a high heat. Cook the meatballs for 2–3 minutes on each side until golden brown all over – you may need to do this in batches depending on the size of your pan. Transfer the meatballs to the tomato sauce and simmer for a further 10 minutes.

4 You can either eat the meatballs straight away or leave them to cool before portioning into labelled freezer bags with the tomato sauce. Ensure to defrost the meatballs fully overnight in the fridge before reheating. If using a microwave, place in a microwavable bowl, cover with a plate or cling film and cook for 3–4 minutes. Stir and heat for a further 3–4 minutes until piping hot all the way through. Times may vary depending on your microwave. If using a saucepan, empty the contents into a medium-sized pan. Add 3–4 tablespoons of water, bring to the boil, then simmer for 5 minutes.

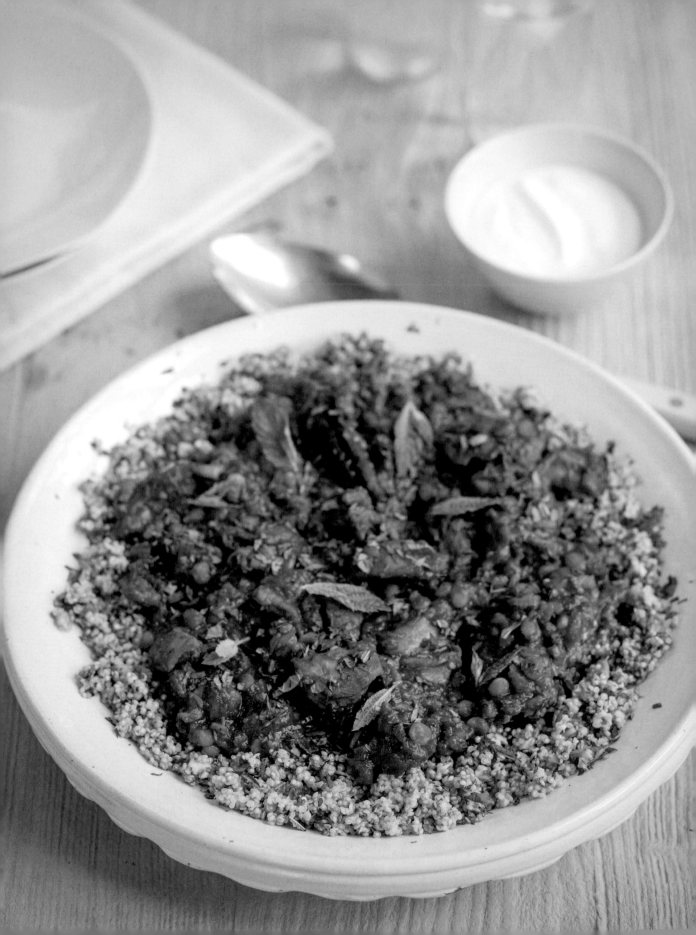

MOROCCAN CHICKEN AND APRICOT TAGINE WITH LENTILS

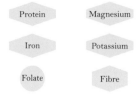

Protein Magnesium

Iron Potassium

Folate Fibre

This is a really flavoursome and aromatic dish minus the heat, which is a good thing you if are breastfeeding, as too much chilli can cause your milk to taste unpleasant. Make a batch while you are on maternity leave – or better still, when people say, 'Let me know if there is anything I can do,' take them up on their offer and send them this recipe! They can then bag it up in individual portions and drop it round, ready to be stashed in your freezer for when the little one arrives. Serve with some couscous, which can be rehydrated in boiling stock or water, some natural yogurt and some fresh coriander. I often also add some chopped pistachios and fresh mint.

PREP TIME 10 MINUTES • COOK TIME 1 HOUR • MAKES 4 PORTIONS

800g free-range chicken thighs, boned and skin removed
1 tbsp harissa paste
1 tbsp rapeseed oil
1 large white onion, peeled and finely sliced
2 garlic cloves, peeled and finely chopped
½ tsp ground cinnamon
1 tsp ground cumin
1 tsp ground coriander
1 tsp ground ginger
1 tsp ground turmeric
1 cinnamon stick
2 tbsp tomato purée
500ml hot chicken stock
125g dried apricots, (look for the darker unsulphured ones)
50g yellow lentils
salt and freshly ground black pepper

TO SERVE
60g couscous (dried weight)
2 tbsp natural yogurt
1 tbsp chopped fresh coriander
1 tbsp chopped pistachio nuts (optional)
1 tbsp chopped fresh mint (optional)

1 Cut the chicken thighs into 4–5cm pieces and coat well with the harissa paste.

2 Heat the oil in a large casserole pan over a medium heat. Add the onion and a large pinch of salt and fry for 4–5 minutes before adding the garlic and marinated chicken. Turn up the heat and cook for 5–6 minutes until the chicken starts to brown.

3 Add the ground cinnamon, cumin, coriander, ginger, turmeric and cinnamon stick. Stir the chicken to coat in the spices and cook for 2–3 minutes before adding the tomato purée and stirring again.

4 Now add the stock, apricots and lentils. Bring to the boil and allow to simmer for 45 minutes.

5 Once cooked, check the seasoning. The tagine can be eaten straight away or allowed to cool before being portioned into labelled freezer bags. Freeze for up to 1 month and ensure you defrost it fully overnight in the fridge before reheating. If using a microwave, place in a microwavable bowl, cover with a plate or cling film and cook for 3–4 minutes, stir and heat for a further 3–4 minutes until piping hot all the way through. Times may vary depending on the strength of your microwave. If using a saucepan, empty the contents of the bag into a medium-sized pan. Add 3–4 tablespoons of water and heat until it starts to boil, then simmer for 5 minutes.

PROVENÇAL CHICKEN STEW

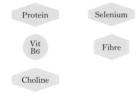

Protein

Selenium

Vit B6

Fibre

Choline

This dish is full of rich tomatoes and plump olives to give you that true taste of the Mediterranean. It also freezes really well and is the perfect nesting dish as it already contains potatoes, so you don't even need to make anything to go with it, although it is great with a big spinach salad or some roasted vegetables, chopped parsley and crusty wholemeal bread.

PREP TIME 10 MINUTES • COOK TIME 45 MINUTES • MAKES 4 PORTIONS

4 large free-range chicken legs, or 4 thighs and 4 drumsticks
4 tbsp rapeseed oil
1 large red onion, peeled and finely chopped
3 garlic cloves, peeled and finely chopped
4 anchovy fillets
2 tsp dried herbes de Provence
1 tsp fennel seeds
1 tbsp tomato purée
200ml white wine
1 x 400g tin chopped tomatoes
300ml hot chicken stock
500g new potatoes, sliced to the thickness of a £1 coin
100g black olives (the small French Nyon variety have a great flavour)
salt and freshly ground black pepper

1 Place a large heavy-based saucepan over a high heat. Season the chicken with salt and pepper. Add half the oil to the pan and cook the chicken for 3–4 minutes on each side until well browned all over – you will probably need to do this in batches. Once browned, remove from the pan and set aside on a plate.

2 Pour the remaining oil into the pan and add the onion, garlic, anchovies, dried herbs and fennel seeds. Cook for 4–5 minutes over a low–medium heat until the onions are soft. Stir regularly to prevent the garlic from burning. Add the tomato purée, stir again and cook for 2–3 minutes before pouring in the wine. Allow the liquid to come to the boil and scrape the bottom of the pan to remove any nice flavoursome bits. Once the wine has reduced by half, add the tomatoes and stock. Bring to the boil.

3 Now, take a stick blender or pour the contents of the saucepan into a food processor and blend until completely smooth. Pour the contents back into the pan. Bring to the boil and add the browned chicken, along with the sliced potatoes and olives. Leave to simmer for 30–40 minutes.

4 Once cooked, remove the stew from the heat and add lots of black pepper. You can eat it straight away or leave it to cool and portion into labelled freezer bags. The stew will keep in the freezer for up to 1 month. Defrost it fully in the fridge overnight before reheating. If using a microwave, place in a microwavable bowl, cover with a plate or cling film and cook for 3–4 minutes, stir and heat for a further 3–4 minutes until piping hot all the way through. Times may vary depending on the strength of your microwave. If using a saucepan, empty the contents of the bag into a medium-sized pan. Add 3–4 tablespoons of water and heat until it starts to boil, then simmer for 5 minutes.

PORTUGUESE PORK AND CHORIZO STEW WITH CHICKPEAS

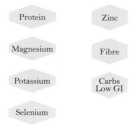

Protein

Magnesium

Potassium

Selenium

Zinc

Fibre

Carbs
Low GI

People often forget that pork is just as good for stewing as lamb, chicken and beef. The natural richness of pork shoulder means it cooks down to become beautifully tender and it stays lovely and moist. I have added chickpeas to this dish to give it some body, and to provide the added energy you will no doubt need during the first few months of having your little one. Even so, I recommend serving this with some nourishing carbohydrates, such as brown rice or bread, to soak up all the delicious juices, and a mixed salad.

PREP TIME 20 MINUTES • COOK TIME 2 HOURS • MAKES 6–8 PORTIONS

2 tbsp rapeseed oil
800g free-range pork shoulder, diced into 2cm pieces
300g cooking chorizo, diced
2 red onions, peeled and finely sliced
3 garlic cloves, peeled and finely chopped
2 tsp smoked paprika
½ tsp chilli powder
2 tsp dried oregano or mixed herbs
2 tbsp tomato purée
400ml hot chicken stock
1 x 400g tin chopped tomatoes
1 tsp runny honey
2 x 400g tins chickpeas, rinsed and drained
1 tbsp sherry vinegar
salt and freshly ground black pepper

TO SERVE
1 tbsp chopped fresh flat-leaf parsley leaves

1 Preheat the oven to 160°C (fan 140°C). Heat the oil in a large casserole dish over a high heat. Season the pork with salt and pepper and, when the oil is hot, add it to the pan. You will probably need to do this in 2 batches so as not to overcrowd the pan. Cook the meat on all sides until well browned. Once the first batch is browned, remove it from the pan, add a little more oil and do the same with the second batch.

2 Return all the browned meat to the pan along with the chorizo and cook over a medium heat for 10 minutes. Now add the onions and garlic, stir well and cook for 5–6 minutes.

3 Add the paprika, chilli, oregano or mixed herbs and the tomato purée. Mix well. Pour in the stock and scrape the bottom of the pan to remove any nice flavoursome bits. Now add the tomatoes, honey, chickpeas and sherry vinegar. Bring to the boil, cover and transfer to the oven for 2 hours.

4 Once the pork is tender, remove the casserole from the oven and either eat at once or leave to cool before portioning into labelled freezer bags. The stew will keep in the freezer for up to 1 month. Defrost fully in the fridge overnight before reheating. If using a microwave, place in a microwavable bowl, cover with a plate or cling film and cook for 3–4 minutes, stir and heat for a further 3–4 minutes until piping hot all the way through. Times may vary depending on your microwave. If using a saucepan, empty the contents of the bag into a medium-sized pan. Add 3–4 tablespoons of water and heat until it starts to boil, then simmer for 5 minutes. Scatter with chopped parsley.

COD AND SWEET POTATO FISH CAKES

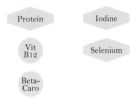

Protein

Iodine

Vit
B12

Selenium

Beta-
Caro

Fish cakes are quick and easy, and making them yourself means you will know exactly what has gone into them. I use sweet potatoes for this recipe as they contain high levels of vitamin A, which can help strengthen a low or recovering immune system. Using sweet potatoes gives the fish cakes a softer texture, as they don't contain the starch that white potatoes do. The addition of spring onions and a little sweetcorn makes these a real treat. Serve with wilted spinach or griddled asparagus and a squeeze of lemon.

PREP TIME 20 MINUTES • COOK TIME 1 HOUR • MAKES 8

3–4 medium sweet potatoes
500g skinless cod fillets or other white fish, cut into small pieces
bunch of spring onions, trimmed and finely chopped
30g fresh coriander leaves, finely chopped
2 tsp Cajun seasoning
1 x 200g tin sweetcorn, drained
salt and freshly ground black pepper

FOR THE COATING
100g plain flour
2 free-range eggs, beaten with 50ml milk
100g polenta, dried wholemeal breadcrumbs or matzo meal

1 Preheat the oven to 200°C (fan 180°C). Place the sweet potatoes on a baking tray and pierce a few times with a knife. Cook for 30–40 minutes, until tender. You can also cook them in the microwave for 8–10 minutes on high if you are in a hurry (or impatient like me), but you will have to cook them 2 at a time as they won't fit in one go. Halve lengthways and leave to cool. Keep the oven on if you are eating the fish cakes immediately.

2 Place the cod fillets, spring onions, coriander, Cajun seasoning and sweetcorn in a food processor and pulse a few times. Season generously with salt and pepper.

3 Scoop the sweet potato flesh into the food processor with the fish mixture, and pulse until all the ingredients are combined but still have a little texture.

4 For the coating, tip the flour into one bowl, the beaten eggs and milk into another, and the polenta, breadcrumbs or meal into a third. Shape the fish cake mixture into 8 patties. Coat each one well in the flour, then shake off the excess and dip into the egg mixture and then the breadcrumbs. Make sure each patty is completely covered. To get a really good coating, dip them back into the egg and then again into the breadcrumbs.

5 Cook the fish cakes on a lightly oiled baking tray in the oven for 20 minutes. Alternatively, freeze the fish cakes on a parchment-lined tray. Make sure they don't touch or they will stick together as they freeze. Once frozen hard, store in labelled freezer bags – I usually put 2 in each bag. When you are ready to cook the fish cakes, preheat the oven to 200°C (fan 180°C). Cook from frozen on a baking tray for 40 minutes.

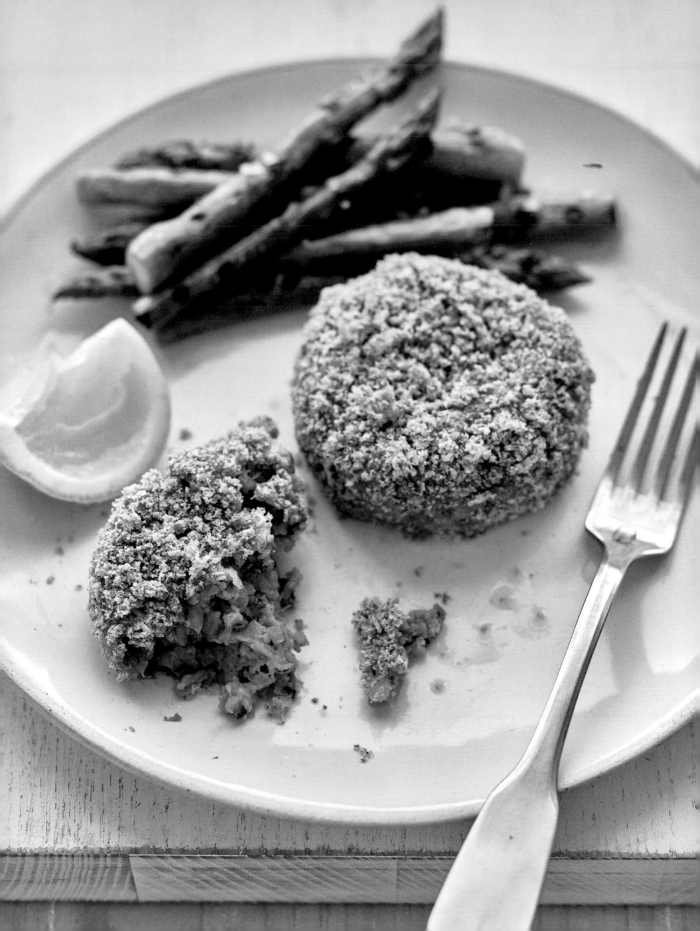

BLACK-EYED BEAN BAKED ENCHILADAS

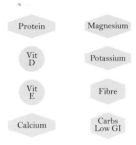

Avocados are a rich source of Vitamin E, which will help your skin to heal after the birth. It will also help with stretch marks on your breasts, which may become noticeable as your milk comes in. This dish is pretty heavy on cheese, and I've done this on purpose. You need extra calories if breastfeeding, and cheese is rich in calcium and vitamin D, both really important, as you will be passing on huge amounts of them to the baby through your breastmilk and need to keep up your supply to prevent brittle bones. Freeze in foil trays, either one 20cm x 30cm or two 10cm x 20cm.

PREP TIME 20 MINUTES • COOK TIME 20 MINUTES, PLUS 35 MINUTES TO REHEAT • MAKES 4 PORTIONS

2 tbsp rapeseed oil
2 red onions, peeled and finely sliced
2 red peppers, deseeded and finely chopped
pinch of chilli flakes
2 garlic cloves, peeled and finely chopped
2 tsp ground cumin
2 tsp Cajun seasoning
1 x 400g tin black-eyed beans, drained
1 x 400g tin pinto beans, drained
1 x 200g tin sweetcorn, drained
500ml tomato passata
8 small soft wholewheat tortillas
2 x 125g balls of mozzarella cheese
30g fresh coriander leaves, chopped
240ml soured cream
150g Cheddar cheese, grated
salt and freshly ground black pepper

TO SERVE
2 avocados
4 lime wedges

1 Preheat the oven to 200°C (fan 180°C) if you plan to eat the enchiladas straight away. Heat the oil in a large frying pan over a medium heat. Add the onions, red peppers, chilli, garlic, cumin and Cajun seasoning. Season well with salt and pepper and cook for 4–5 minutes. Add the beans and sweetcorn to the pan and mix well, mashing the beans slightly using either the back of a fork or a potato masher. Mix through 4 tablespoons of the passata, then transfer the mixture to a bowl to cool slightly.

2 Lay the tortillas out on a board and divide the cooled bean mixture between them. Now tear over the mozzarella cheese and sprinkle with the coriander. Roll the tortillas up carefully like a cigar and lay them into the tray(s). Pour over the remaining passata and dot over the soured cream, then top with the grated Cheddar cheese.

3 The enchiladas can now be covered tightly with cling film and frozen for up to 1 month. Remember to label them so you know what they are and the date they were made. To reheat, defrost them fully overnight in the fridge before cooking in a preheated 200°C (fan 180°C) oven for 35 minutes, until bubbling. Alternatively, cook immediately in the oven for 35 minutes. Serve with mashed avocado and a wedge of fresh lime.

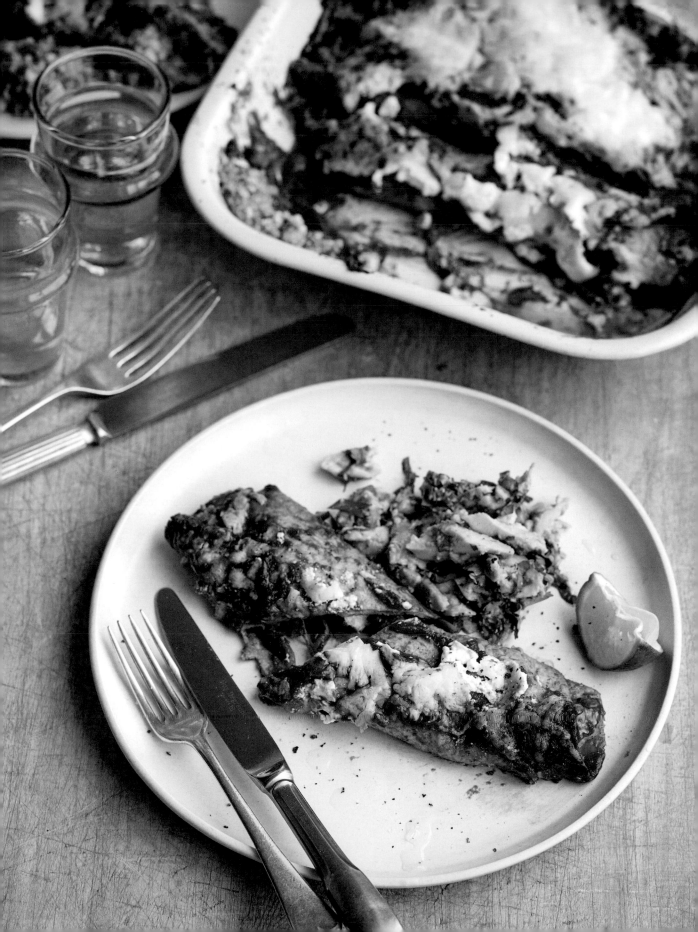

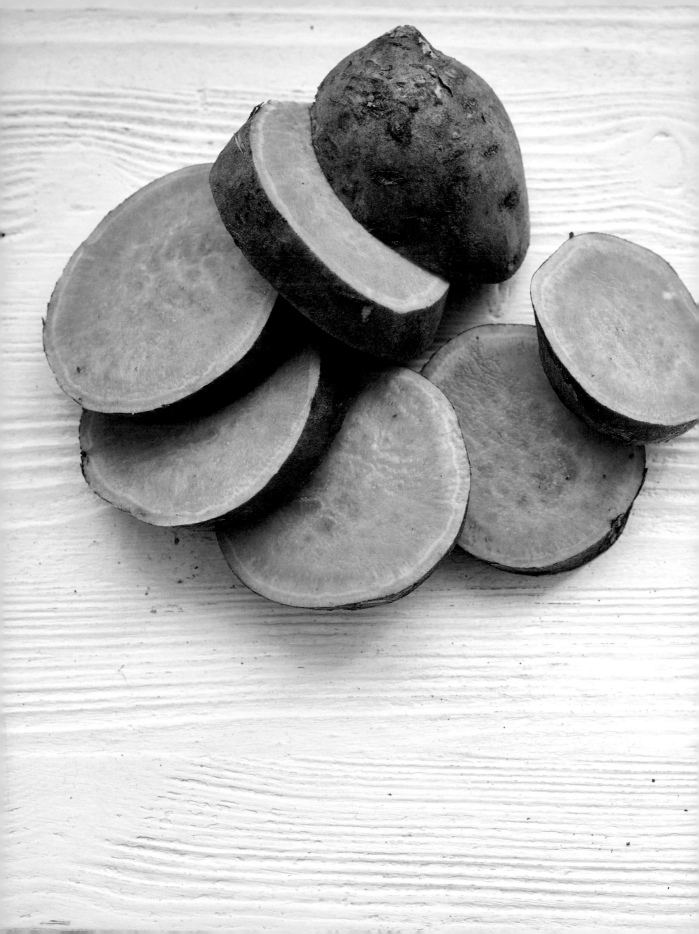

SOUPS

Soups are great throughout all stages of pregnancy. From about 24 weeks I started to find that I felt full really quickly, and soups offered a great alternative to larger main meals.

I also love the idea of throwing lots of really fresh, wholesome and nutritious ingredients into a pan and seeing what comes out once cooked. I don't like wasting food, and with soups, you can pretty much throw in anything that might not otherwise get eaten. Make a big batch to take to work in a flask for lunch.

Soup freezes really well, so have some in the freezer for the nights when you really don't fancy cooking. I'd also recommend stocking up just before baby is born, as soup is a great meal to eat one-handed!

Try not to overcook your vegetables, especially the green ones, to ensure that they keep their colour and therefore their vital minerals and vitamins. Always add greens right at the end of cooking. Also, buy 'Pour and Store' bags; these are available from all supermarkets and make storing soups and others sauces in the freezer really easy.

Take stock

Making soups using a stock cube is absolutely fine and will of course save you time. But if you are the type who doesn't like waste, try saving your vegetable trimmings, odd bits of veg that have seen better days and leftover meat bones and to make your own stock. This can then be frozen in portions and used in soups (or stews and gravy) as and when needed. Here are some basic instructions for making simple chicken or vegetable stock. Of course, you can use any leftover veg or trimmings you already have – apart from potatoes and any vegetables that will break down too much and make your stock cloudy.

CHICKEN STOCK

MAKES 2–3 LITRES

Chop 1 carrot, 1 celery stick, 1 onion and 1 leek into roughly 6cm chunks. Put in a large saucepan (or stockpot) with any trimmings, 2 bay leaves, 6 parsley stalks and 6 peppercorns. Add the carcass from a leftover chicken (skin removed) and cover with cold water. Bring to the boil over a high heat, then use a ladle to skim off any of the scum that has gathered on the surface. Reduce the heat to low and simmer for 4–5 hours. Cover with a lid if you have one and keep topping up with water. Remove any more impurities that come to the surface. When it has simmered, strain the stock into a clean pot through a sieve. Chill and then either use within a couple of days or freeze for up to 3 months.

VEGETABLE STOCK

The method is the same as above, but you will need to up your veggies. Use 2 carrots, 2 celery sticks, 2 onions, 1 leek, 2 bay leaves, 6 parsley stalks and 6 peppercorns.

CAULIFLOWER AND ALMOND SOUP

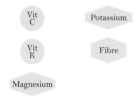

Vit C

Potassium

Vit K

Fibre

Magnesium

This soup is velvety smooth and very luxurious. Cauliflower tends to get overlooked as a vegetable but it has an amazing nutty flavour which pairs fabulously with almonds. This soup is rich in both magnesium and potassium – two of the most important minerals our bodies need to maintain a healthy pregnancy and good fertility.

PREP TIME 10 MINUTES • COOK TIME 20 MINUTES • MAKES 1.5 LITRES

2 tbsp rapeseed oil
1 large white onion, peeled and finely sliced
2 garlic cloves, peeled and finely chopped
1 cauliflower head, cut into 2 cm pieces, stalk and all
2 thyme sprigs, leaves picked
1 litre hot vegetable or chicken stock
100g whole blanched almonds
salt and freshly ground black pepper

TO SERVE
4 tsp flaked almonds, toasted
2 tbsp extra virgin olive oil or walnut oil

1 Heat the oil in a large saucepan over a medium heat. Add the onion and cook for 5–6 minutes, then stir the garlic and cauliflower into the onion. Add the thyme leaves, cover, and cook for 5 minutes, until softened, stirring occasionally. Add a pinch of salt and pepper. Now add the stock and almonds, cover and cook until the cauliflower is very tender. This will take about 15 minutes.

2 Once cooked, transfer to a blender (you may need to do this in 2 batches) and blitz until silky smooth. This can also be done using a stick blender. Season to taste.

3 If you wish to keep the soup for later, cool completely before pouring into labelled freezer bags and storing in the freezer for up to 1 month. Defrost overnight in the fridge before reheating. Alternatively, cool and store in an airtight container in the fridge for 3–4 days. Make sure the soup is piping hot before serving; this can be done in a saucepan or in the microwave.

4 Serve sprinkled with the toasted flaked almonds and a drizzle of olive oil or walnut oil.

PEA, COURGETTE AND MINT SOUP

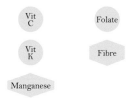

Vit C

Folate

Vit K

Fibre

Manganese

The vibrant green colour of this soup lets you know it's full of goodness, and it will make you feel instantly better the second you taste a mouthful. Hormones and carrying a baby around for 9 months can make your body temperature rise while pregnant, so I often served this soup chilled. Additionally, by not overheating, you won't destroy too many of the soup's nutrients and vitamins.

PREP TIME 10 MINUTES • COOK TIME 15 MINUTES • MAKES 1.5 LITRES

2 tbsp rapeseed oil
1 large white onion, peeled and finely sliced
2 garlic cloves, peeled and finely chopped
1 litre hot vegetable or chicken stock
300g frozen petits pois or garden peas
2 large courgettes, trimmed and grated
200g baby leaf spinach
20 fresh mint leaves
salt and freshly ground black pepper

1 Heat the oil in a large saucepan over a medium heat, then add the onion and cook for 5–6 minutes. Add the garlic and stock and bring to the boil. Season with a little salt and pepper. Once boiling, add the peas, courgettes, spinach and mint leaves. Cook for 2 minutes until the spinach is wilted.

2 Remove from the heat and leave to cool before pouring the soup into a blender and blitzing until smooth (you may need to do this in 2 batches). You can also do this with a stick blender. Either eat straightaway or reheat in the saucepan.

3 If you wish to keep the soup for later, leave it to cool completely before pouring into labelled freezer bags and storing in the freezer for up to 1 month. Defrost overnight in the fridge before reheating. Alternatively, cool and store in an airtight container in the fridge for 3–4 days. Make sure to reheat the soup thoroughly before serving (or cooling again if you would like to eat it chilled); this can be done in a saucepan or in the microwave.

PUMPKIN, COCONUT AND GINGER SOUP

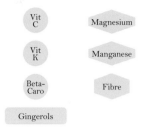

Vit C · Magnesium · Vit K · Manganese · Beta-Caro · Fibre · Gingerols

This soup is smooth, creamy and wholesome. The gently warming ginger not only helps to counteract sickness but also does wonders for a low immune system in a tired and hard-working mum or mum-to-be.

PREP TIME 15 MINUTES • COOK TIME 30 MINUTES • MAKES 1.5 LITRES

2 tbsp rapeseed oil
1 butternut squash
 or 500g pumpkin,
 peeled, deseeded and
 diced into 2cm pieces
1 white onion, peeled
 and finely chopped
1 celery stick, finely
 chopped
1 garlic clove, peeled
 and finely chopped
1½ tsp ground ginger
5cm piece fresh ginger,
 peeled and finely
 chopped
200ml coconut milk
1 litre hot chicken
 or vegetable stock

TO SERVE
2 tbsp pumpkin seeds

1 Heat the oil in a large saucepan over a low heat. Add the diced vegetables and garlic, along with a pinch of salt, and allow to sweat for 6–8 minutes. Add the ground and fresh ginger and cook for a further minute before adding the coconut milk and stock.

2 Bring to the boil, then reduce the heat, cover with a lid and simmer until the vegetables are tender and falling apart. This should take about 20 minutes.

3 Once cooked, remove the soup from the heat and leave to cool a little before pouring into a blender and blitzing until smooth (you may need to do this in 2 batches). You can also do this using a stick blender.

4 You can now store the soup either in the fridge or freezer. Allow to cool completely before pouring into an airtight container and keeping in the fridge for 3–4 days, or pour into labelled freezer bags and store in the freezer for up to 1 month. Defrost overnight in the fridge before reheating. Ensure the soup is piping hot before you serve it; this can be done in a saucepan or in the microwave.

5 Add a sprinkling of pumpkin seeds before serving for some extra texture.

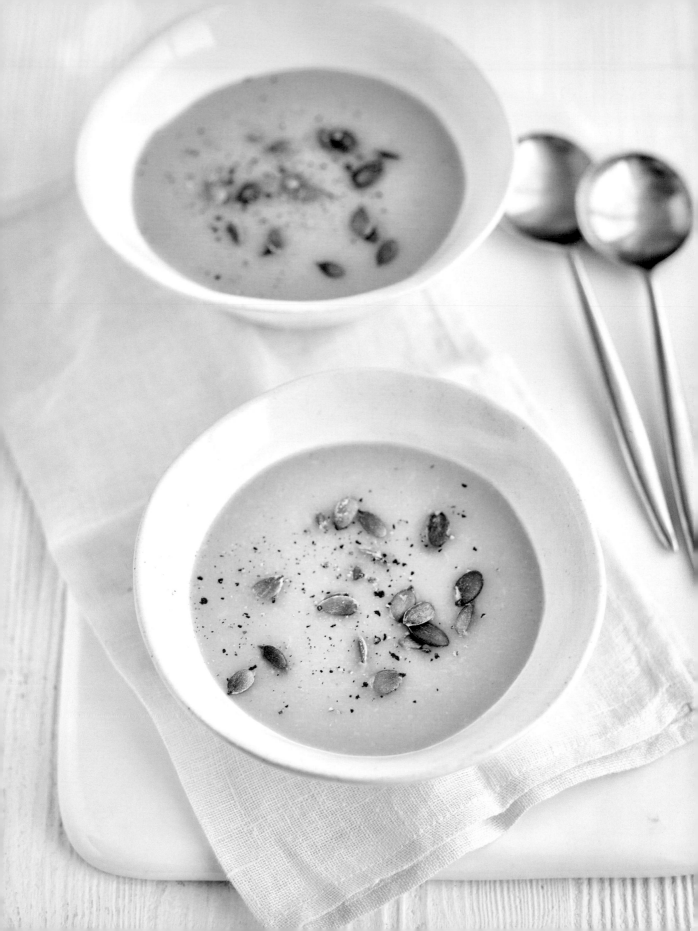

RED LENTIL, CUMIN AND CARROT SOUP

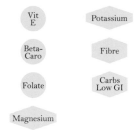

Vit E

Potassium

Beta-Caro

Fibre

Folate

Carbs Low GI

Magnesium

This soup will slowly release energy throughout the day, leaving you feeling nice and full. It is also a good source of folate and fibre. Carrots have a natural sweetness that really balances the nuttiness of red lentils, and warming cumin is the perfect bridge between the two ingredients. I often make this soup if I'm not feeling 100 per cent; the cumin is great if you are feeling a little congested or off-colour.

PREP TIME 10 MINUTES • COOK TIME 30 MINUTES • MAKES 1.5 LITRES

2 tbsp rapeseed oil
2 tsp cumin seeds
1 large white onion, peeled and finely sliced
2 garlic cloves, peeled and finely chopped
140g red lentils
600g carrots, peeled and roughly chopped
1 tsp ground ginger
1.25 litres hot chicken or vegetable stock
salt and freshly ground black pepper

TO SERVE
2 tbsp natural yogurt
2 tbsp pumpkin or sunflower seeds

1 Heat the oil in a large saucepan over a medium heat. Add the cumin seeds and cook for 1 minute before adding the onion and cooking for another 5–6 minutes. Stir in the garlic, lentils, carrots and ginger. Pour in the stock and bring to the boil. Season with a little salt and pepper. Once boiling, reduce the heat and simmer until the carrots and lentils are tender. This will take about 20 minutes.

2 Once cooked, remove the soup from the heat and leave to cool a little before pouring into a blender and blitzing until smooth (you may need to do this in 2 batches). You can also do this using a stick blender.

3 You can now store the soup either in the fridge or freezer. Allow to cool completely before pouring into an airtight container and keeping in the fridge for 3–4 days, or pour into labelled freezer bags and store in the freezer for up to 1 month. Defrost overnight in the fridge before reheating. Ensure the soup is piping hot before you serve it; this can be done in a saucepan or in the microwave.

4 I like to serve mine with a spoonful of natural yogurt and a sprinkle of pumpkin or sunflower seeds.

SPINACH, KALE AND WATERCRESS SOUP

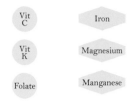

Vit C

Vit K

Folate

Iron

Magnesium

Manganese

This soup contains huge amounts of iron and folate, both of which are essential for maintaining good energy levels and healthy blood. They can also help protect against developing infections or anaemia.

It can literally be made in minutes and can be eaten hot or cold. Perfect for a busy mum-to-be who needs a quick green pick-me-up. Remember that the longer you cook vegetables for, the fewer nutrients they will contain, so quick cooking is essential to save time and, more importantly, to ensure you get the maximum goodness available.

PREP TIME 5 MINUTES • COOK TIME 15 MINUTES • MAKES 1.5 LITRES

2 tbsp rapeseed oil
1 white onion, peeled and finely sliced
2 garlic cloves, peeled and finely chopped
1 large potato, peeled and finely diced
1 litre hot vegetable or chicken stock
200g kale
200g baby leaf spinach
200g watercress
salt and freshly ground black pepper

TO SERVE
4 tsp natural yogurt
2 tbsp extra virgin olive oil

1 Heat the oil in a large saucepan or casserole pan over a low heat. Add the onion, garlic and potato and cook for 5–6 minutes. Season with a little salt and pepper. Once the onion is soft, add the stock and bring to the boil, then simmer until the potato is completely soft; this should take about 10 minutes. Add the kale, spinach and watercress, and cook for 30 seconds to 1 minute until everything is wilted.

2 Remove the soup from the heat and leave to cool a little before pouring into a blender and blitzing until smooth (you may need to do this in 2 batches). You can also do this using a stick blender.

3 You can now store the soup either in the fridge or freezer. Allow to cool completely before pouring into an airtight container and keeping in the fridge for 3–4 days, or pour into labelled freezer bags and store in the freezer for up to 1 month. Defrost overnight in the fridge before reheating. Ensure the soup is piping hot before you serve it; this can be done in a saucepan or in the microwave.

4 Add a spoonful of yogurt to each bowl and drizzle with olive oil before serving.

GREEN MINESTRONE

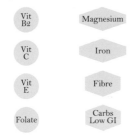

Vit B2	Magnesium
Vit C	Iron
Vit E	Fibre
Folate	Carbs Low GI

Eating lots of greenery is great for you and baby, and this soup is surely going to put a big tick in that folate and iron box. Green vegetables are also a really good source of vitamin E, which will do wonders for your skin and could even help prevent stretch marks. It's really important to remember, however, that all nutrients and vitamins are very precious and can easily be destroyed by overcooking, so quick cooking and eating al dente is always advised.

PREP TIME 15 MINUTES • COOK TIME 20 MINUTES • MAKE 1.5 LITRES

2 tbsp rapeseed oil
1 white onion, peeled and finely diced
1 leek, trimmed and finely diced
2 garlic cloves, peeled and finely chopped
½ fennel bulb, trimmed and finely diced
1 celery stick, finely chopped
1.5 litres hot chicken or vegetable stock
200g wholegrain giant couscous or baby pasta
2 courgettes, trimmed and grated
2 spring onions, trimmed and sliced
2 handfuls of petits pois, fresh or frozen
1 handful of broad beans, fresh or frozen
6–8 baby asparagus spears, trimmed and halved lengthways
salt and freshly ground black pepper

TO SERVE
4 tsp green pesto or Emerald Pesto (page 76)
20g Parmesan cheese, grated

1 Heat the oil in a large saucepan or casserole pan over a low heat. Add the onion, leek, garlic, fennel and celery, and cook for 5–6 minutes until the vegetables start to soften. Now add the stock, increase the heat and bring to the boil. Season with a little salt and lots of pepper. Reduce the heat and simmer for a few minutes before adding the couscous or baby pasta. Cook for 10 minutes or until just tender. Now add the courgettes, spring onions, peas, broad beans and baby asparagus. Simmer for 1–2 minutes before turning off the heat.

2 If you don't want to eat the soup straight away, you can store it either in the fridge or freezer. Allow to cool completely before pouring into an airtight container and keeping in the fridge for 3–4 days, or pour into labelled freezer bags and store in the freezer for up to 1 month. Defrost overnight in the fridge before reheating. Ensure the soup is piping hot before you serve it; this can be done in a saucepan or in the microwave.

3 Serve with a spoonful of pesto and a sprinkling of Parmesan.

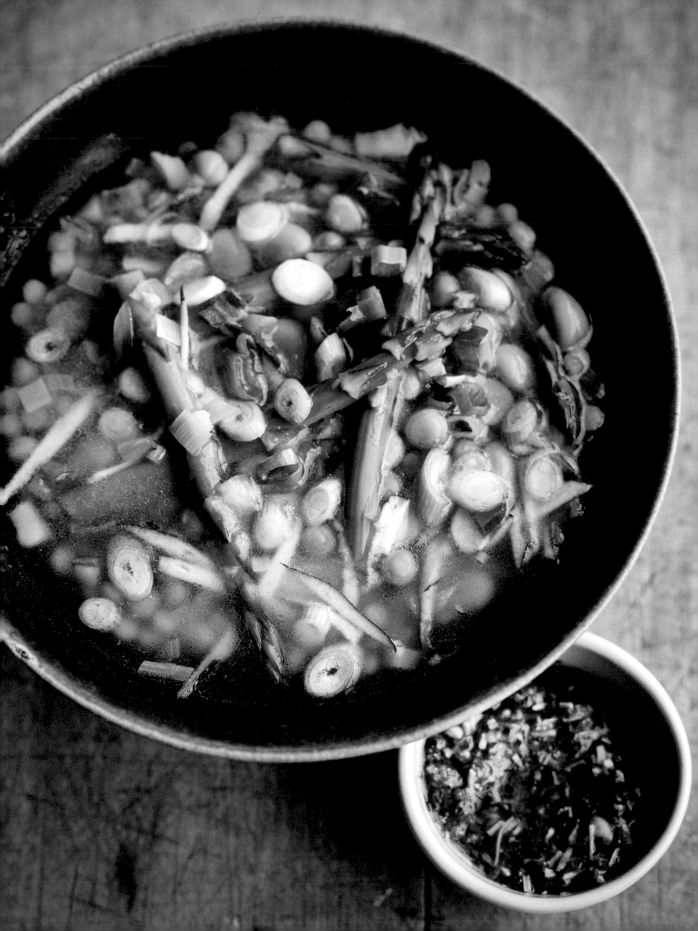

COD, CHICKPEA AND SWEET POTATO SOUP

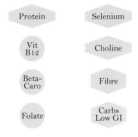

Protein • Selenium
Vit B12 • Choline
Beta-Caro • Fibre
Folate • Carbs Low GI

This is halfway between a soup and a stew. Cod is rich in selenium, which can improve fertility (so good if you are reading this recipe before falling pregnant). It also has antioxidant qualities which protect cells from damage in both mum and baby. It can be made in advance and kept in the fridge (for up to 3 days), ready to reheat whenever you fancy a warming bowlful. Leave out the chilli if you're suffering from heartburn or indigestion.

PREP TIME 15 MINUTES • COOK TIME 20 MINUTES • SERVES 4

2 tbsp rapeseed oil
1 large red onion, peeled and finely chopped
2 garlic cloves, peeled and finely chopped
1 tsp ground cumin
½ tsp fennel seeds
1 tsp smoked paprika
½ tsp chilli flakes (optional)
1 tbsp tomato purée
1.5 litre hot chicken or vegetable stock
2 large sweet potatoes, peeled and chopped into 2cm pieces
1 x 400g tin chickpeas, rinsed and drained
400g skinless cod fillets, cut into 2cm pieces
salt and freshly ground black pepper

TO SERVE
2–3 tbsp flat-leaf parsley or coriander, finely chopped
1 tbsp sunflower seeds
1 tbsp flaked almonds
4 tsp natural yogurt

1 Heat the oil in a large casserole pan over a medium heat and add the onion, garlic, cumin, fennel seeds, smoked paprika and chilli flakes (if using). Cook for 3–4 minutes, stirring all the time. Add the tomato purée and cook for a further 2 minutes. Pour in the stock and bring to the boil. Season with salt and pepper, and add the sweet potato. Lower the heat and simmer for 10–15 minutes, until tender, before adding the chickpeas and cod. Cook for 5–6 minutes before turning off the heat.

2 If you are freezing the soup, leave it to cool completely before portioning into labelled freezer bags. It will keep for up to 1 month in the freezer. Defrost it overnight in the fridge before reheating. You can also cool the soup and store it in an airtight container in the fridge for up to 3 days. Reheat it gently but thoroughly in a saucepan or in the microwave.

3 Before serving, gently stir through the chopped herbs, then sprinkle over the sunflower seeds and almonds, and add a spoonful of yogurt to each bowl.

CHICKEN, KALE AND BARLEY HEALING BROTH

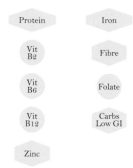

Protein · Iron · Vit B2 · Fibre · Vit B6 · Folate · Vit B12 · Carbs Low GI · Zinc

Chicken soup or broth made from bones has been proven to heal your gut, promoting healthy digestion, as well as being an anti-inflammatory, good for swollen ankles and feet. It inhibits infection and so helps maintain a healthy immune system, and is great for bones and joint health due to its high amounts of calcium and magnesium.

I'm not going to try to reinvent the wheel here. This is my version of chicken soup, the one I love and which always makes me feel better.

PREP TIME 10 MINUTES • COOK TIME 1½ HOURS • MAKES 1.5 LITRES

1 x 1–1.2kg free-range chicken
1 white onion, peeled and halved
2 bay leaves
2 thyme sprigs
1.5 litres hot water, or enough to cover the chicken
80g barley
2 large carrots, peeled and finely diced
1 celery stick, finely diced
1 leek, trimmed and finely diced
3 handfuls of kale
salt and freshly ground black pepper

1 Place the chicken, onion, bay leaves and thyme in deep casserole pan. Pour in enough water to cover the chicken and bring to the boil with a large pinch of salt. Once boiling, turn the heat down to a simmer and cook gently for 1 hour. Meanwhile, place the barley in a small bowl, cover with cold water and soak for 20 minutes. Once soaked, drain well.

2 When the chicken is cooked, carefully remove it from the broth and leave to cool. Strain the broth through a fine sieve into a clean pan to remove any herbs, onion and bits of the chicken that may have come loose. Place the strained stock back on the stove and add the carrots, celery, leeks and soaked barley. Bring to the boil and cook until the vegetables and barley are tender. This should take about 20 minutes.

3 While the broth is simmering, shred the chicken. It will be hot, so I recommend you wear clean rubber gloves for this stage. You may not want to use all the chicken – I think the leg meat tastes best in this broth, and I often keep the breast meat for a sandwich or stir-fry the next day. Add the shredded chicken to the simmering broth along with the kale. Season with pepper and allow the kale to wilt for 2 minutes. Remove from the heat and serve.

4 If you want to save your broth to eat later, wait for it to cool completely before storing it in labelled freezer bags. It will keep in the freezer for up to 1 month. Defrost it overnight in the fridge before reheating. Alternatively, you can store the broth in an airtight container in the fridge for 3–4 days. Make sure you reheat it thoroughly before serving.

PORK, GINGER AND BUCKWHEAT SOBA NOODLE SOUP

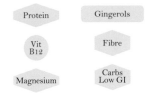

Protein

Vit B12

Magnesium

Gingerols

Fibre

Carbs Low GI

This soup is great during the first trimester of pregnancy as it may help to keep your nausea at bay. Healing qualities come from the ginger, which is an anti-inflammatory and has anti-nausea properties which will help with any swelling you are experiencing as well as morning sickness. Leave out the chilli if you're suffering from heartburn or indigestion.

PREP TIME 15 MINUTES • COOK TIME 25 MINUTES • SERVES 2

200g pork fillet
1 tbsp rapeseed oil
2 tsp Chinese five-spice powder
1 litre hot chicken or vegetable stock
7cm piece fresh ginger, peeled and cut into matchsticks
1 garlic clove, peeled and finely chopped
½ red chilli, deseeded and sliced (optional)
2 tbsp light soy sauce
200g buckwheat soba noodles (or wholewheat noodles)
2 pak choi heads, cut into wedges
2 spring onions, trimmed and finely sliced
1 handful of bean sprouts
10g fresh coriander leaves
salt

TO SERVE
2 lime wedges

1 Preheat the oven to 210°C (fan 190°C). Start by rubbing the pork fillet with the oil and the Chinese five-spice powder. Season with a little salt and place on a baking sheet. Roast for 15–20 minutes, depending on the thickness of the pork.

2 While the pork is cooking, make the broth. Pour the stock into a saucepan and add the ginger, garlic, chilli (if using) and soy sauce. Bring to the boil, then reduce the heat and simmer for 5 minutes. Add the noodles, pak choi and half the spring onions, and cook for a further 4–5 minutes until everything is tender. Remove from the heat.

3 By now the pork should be just about ready. Remove from the oven and allow it to rest for 5–10 minutes before carving it into thin slices. Spoon the noodles and pak choi into large serving bowls and top with half a handful of bean sprouts. Add 4–5 slices of pork per bowl, plus the fresh coriander. Ladle over the hot broth, scatter over the rest of the spring onions, and serve with a wedge of lime.

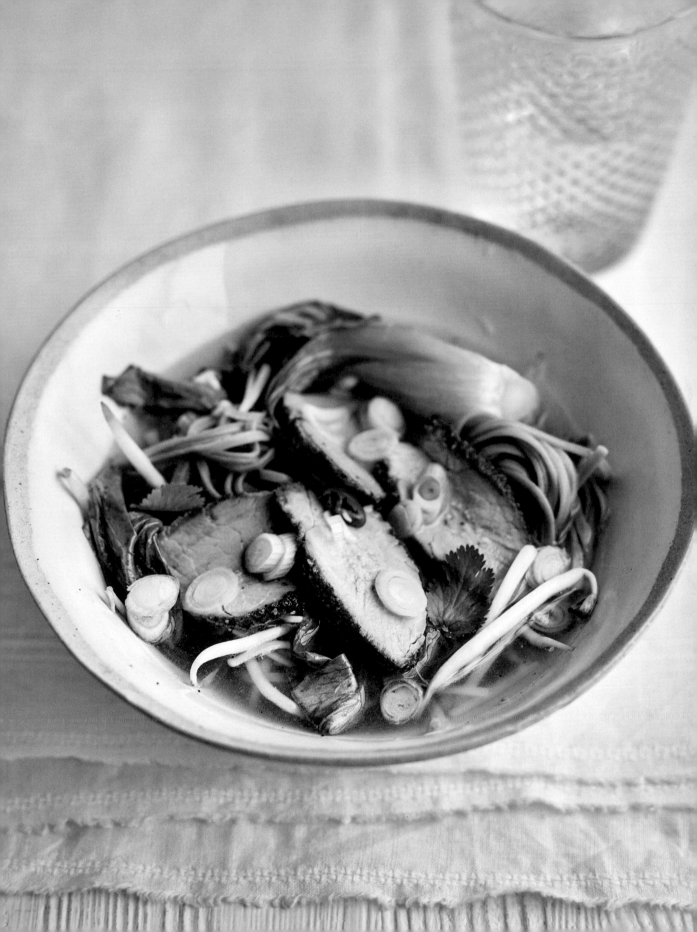

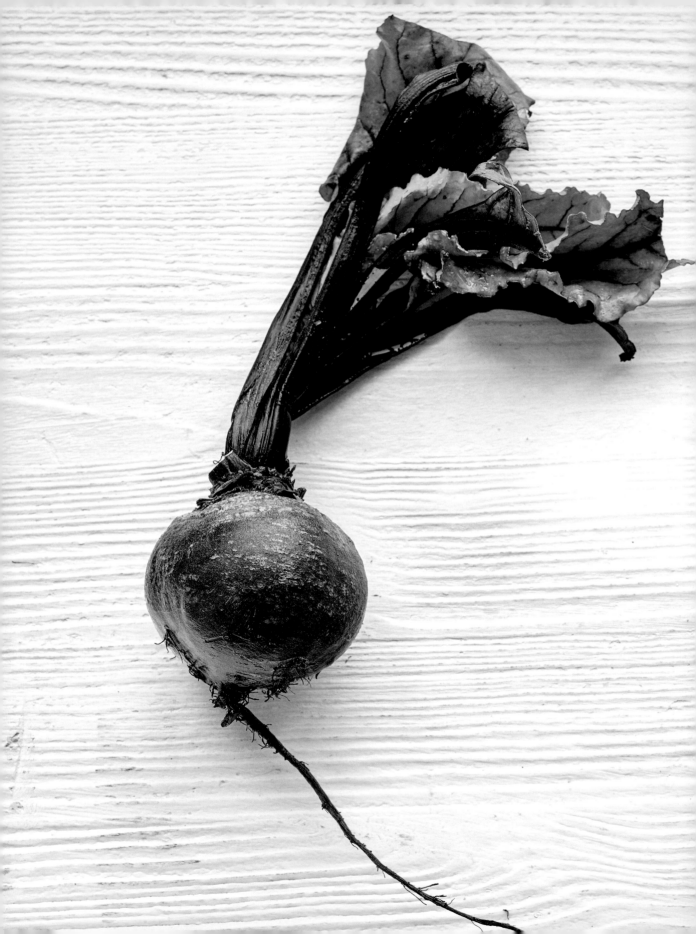

HEALTHY SNACKS

During your pregnancy, especially in the first and third trimesters, it's quite likely that you will only want to eat little and often. In the first trimester, small meals and snacks will help to regulate your blood-sugar levels and hopefully keep morning sickness at bay. In the third trimester, because baby is taking up so much space in your abdomen, your stomach doesn't have enough room to accommodate large meals. Heartburn can also make big meals hard to manage in one sitting.

Some women also find that they seem to be permanently hungry during their pregnancy, and it's easy to be tempted into eating unhealthy snacks like sugary and fatty cakes and biscuits between meals. These will not only cause big sugar peaks and dips, which can lead to you feeling lethargic and sluggish, but your digestion will also suffer from lack of fibre and excess sugar and salt. Although we all need a treat now and then, it's a good idea to try to make them healthy whenever you can.

The snacks in this chapter are perfectly suited to the little-and-often approach. They are great if you are heading out on a commute and fear that sickness may strike, or have a long day head and need some homemade treats in your handbag. Many of these snacks can be prepared a week or so in advance and kept in the cupboard, so you can feel confident that you are giving your baby much-needed nutrients as well as satisfying your hunger. Of course, these snacks can also be enjoyed before pregnancy, when preparing your body for the possibility of carrying a baby, and also after the birth, when your mealtimes might be a bit erratic and you need to keep tiredness and hunger in check. Rich in vital vitamins and minerals, these recipes are designed to give you a boost of energy and a proper dose of the real 'good stuff' to prepare, nourish and recharge you for the days, weeks and months ahead.

Keep hunger at bay

While pregnant you may find that you have a constant need to nibble due to that rapidly growing baby, or maybe you feel sick quite a lot of the time and don't fancy anything big to eat at all. Whichever of those camps you fall into, or if you are somewhere in the middle, this chapter is going to be an important one. Here are some more top snacking tips:

* Healthy snacking can help control blood-sugar levels. Snacking on healthy treats will help stabilise your blood sugars and keep you on a level keel, preventing those peaks and crashes.

* Morning sickness can hit at any time throughout pregnancy, especially during the first trimester. By avoiding letting yourself get too hungry, you can help prevent those intense periods of sickness.

* Try eating a few snacks first thing in the morning, about 15 minutes before getting up. This may help take the edge of the sickness and give you time to get ready before you eat a proper breakfast.

* Have a few homemade snacks in your handbag for your journey to work, just in case you get a bout of sickness or pang of hunger on the commute.

* Research also suggests that counting while chewing or sucking can help take your mind off feeling sick. Try this with an oat cake or even some peppermint chewing gum.

* Stay well hydrated at all times – sometimes hunger is mistaken for thirst.

APPLE CHIPS

These are quick to make and are guaranteed to taste much better than any that you might find in a shop. In all honesty, these apple crisps aren't bursting with goodness, except for being a very good source of vitamin C and fibre, but they are much healthier than any processed snack you might crave, are cheap to prepare and are really delicious for the whole family.

PREP TIME 15 MINUTES • COOK TIME 30 MINUTES • MAKES 4 PORTIONS

4 apples
4 tbsp runny honey
2 tsp ground cinnamon

1 Preheat the oven to 160°C and line 2–3 baking trays with parchment. (Do not use the fan setting or else the chips will blow around in the oven.)

2 Slice the apples as thinly as you can, either using a mandolin (being very careful, as the blade is very sharp) or a sharp knife, leaving the skin on. Lay the apple slices on the prepared baking trays, making sure they are not touching.

3 Heat the honey and cinnamon in a small saucepan until very runny. Brush each apple slice with a little of the honey and cinnamon mixture, then bake in the oven for 15 minutes. Remove the trays from the oven, turn over the slices and brush them with the remaining honey. Return to the oven for a further 15 minutes. You may want to switch the trays around to ensure even cooking.

4 Once the apple crisps are slightly golden and firm to the touch, remove them from the oven and leave to cool on a wire rack. They can be stored in an airtight container for 2–3 days, ready for instant snacking.

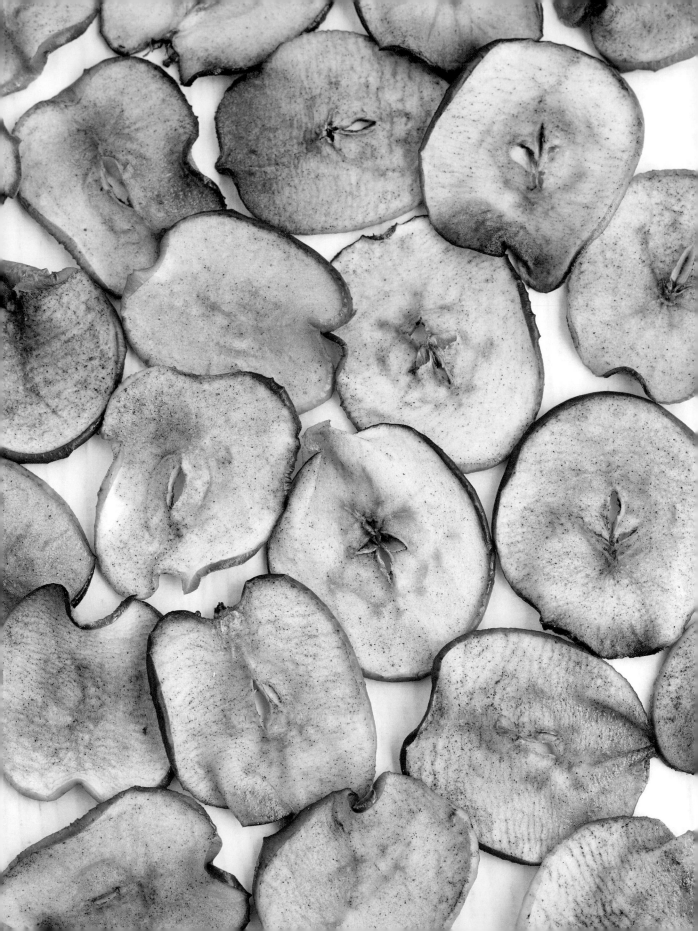

SESAME AND PARMESAN KALE CRISPS

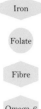

Iron

Folate

Fibre

Omega-6

Kale crisps really do satisfy that urge to eat something crunchy and a little salty, which is of course the main reason most of us head for the crisp packet. I can promise you that the second you open your homemade packet at work, your colleagues will flock, both out of curiosity and because they will wish they had made a batch for themselves, so feel free to share the recipe.

Once made into crisps, the kale retains a nice amount of iron and folate, and will also add fibre to your diet.

PREP TIME 10 MINUTES • COOK TIME 15–20 MINUTES • MAKES 4–5 PORTIONS

1 large bunch of curly kale
3–4 tbsp rapeseed oil
2 tsp sesame seeds
    (black and white)
20g Parmesan
    cheese, grated
1–2 tsp ground cumin or
    smoked paprika (optional)

1 Preheat the oven to 140°C and line 2–3 baking trays with parchment. (Do not use the fan setting or else the chips will blow around in the oven.)

2 Prepare the kale by tearing or cutting the curly leaves away from the woody stalks. Cut each leaf into bite-sized pieces, about 5–6cm each.

3 Place the leaves in a bowl and drizzle over the oil, then add the sesame seeds and Parmesan cheese, and mix well. Lay the coated kale on the prepared baking trays, separating the leaves out as much as possible, and sprinkle over the sesame seeds and Parmesan left in the bowl. Ground cumin or smoked paprika also makes a great addition at this stage.

4 Bake in the oven for 15–20 minutes, turning the kale once during cooking and swapping the trays around to ensure even cooking. Once the kale has dried out and gone crispy, remove from the oven and leave to cool completely before storing. I prefer to store the crisps in small portions in sandwich bags, ready to eat as and when. This tasty snack will stay crisp and last for up to 1 week in an airtight container.

FENNEL AND FLAXSEED OATCAKES

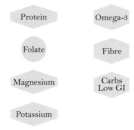

Protein

Folate

Magnesium

Potassium

Omega-3

Fibre

Carbs
Low GI

I know you can buy oatcakes in the supermarket, but once you have made these, you won't want to buy them ever again. The beauty of making your own oatcakes is knowing exactly what has gone into them, ensuring you have complete control over what you and your baby are eating. I have chosen fennel seeds and flaxseed to flavour these oatcakes, to aid digestion and boost omega-3 levels.

PREP TIME 15 MINUTES • COOK TIME 25 MINUTES • MAKES 16

225g rolled porridge oats
75g wholemeal flour,
    plus extra for rolling
2 tbsp milled flaxseed
1½ tsp fennel seeds,
    crushed or gently
    chopped
70g cold butter, cut into
    small cubes, plus extra
    for greasing
1 tsp bicarbonate of soda
80–100ml just-boiled water

1 Preheat the oven to 200°C (fan 180°C). Mix the oats with the flour, flaxseed and fennel seeds in a large bowl. Add the butter and, using your fingers, rub into the flour until the mixture resembles breadcrumbs. Add the bicarbonate of soda and slowly add the hot water. Mix to form a dough – you may not need all the water.

2 Dust your work surface generously with flour and turn out the dough. Lightly knead it into a ball. Using a floured rolling pin, roll out the dough to a thickness of ½cm. Using a 5–6cm cutter, cut out as many oatcakes as you can. Reroll the excess and cut out more if there is lots of dough left over.

3 Lightly butter a non-stick baking tray and carefully lift the oatcakes onto it. Bake in the oven for about 25 minutes, until golden. Leave to cool completely on a wire rack before storing in an airtight container, ready for serving or snacking as and when you wish. They will keep in an airtight container for up to 1 week.

SWEET AND SALTY MUNCHY SEEDS AND NUTS

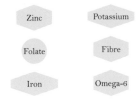

Zinc

Folate

Iron

Potassium

Fibre

Omega-6

My handbag is still scattered with the remains of these tasty treats. They are so moreish and really help to keep the sickness at bay during the first trimester. They are also great to have as a little pick-me-up throughout pregnancy and contain lots of the essential vitamins and minerals that you and your baby need. They are also very good after birth and during preconception as a healthy snack. You can buy similar snacks, but it's so much cheaper to make your own. Fill 5–6 sandwich bags with individual portions and have them ready to go, as and when you need them. Just remember to seal the bag… I didn't!

PREP TIME 5 MINUTES • COOK TIME 15 MINUTES • MAKES 5 X 100G BAGS

2 free-range egg whites
1½ tbsp runny honey
100g whole almonds
75g macadamia nuts
100g whole walnuts
100g whole pecans
50g pumpkin seeds
25g sesame seeds
50g sunflower seeds
1 tsp ground cinnamon
1 tsp ground cumin
1 tsp flaked sea salt

1 Preheat the oven to 180°C (fan 160°C) and line a baking tray with parchment.

2 Mix the egg whites with the honey. Pour all the nuts and seeds into a large bowl and pour over the egg white and honey mixture. Stir well, coating all the nuts and seeds, before adding the spices and salt. Mix again.

3 Spoon the mixture evenly onto the prepared baking tray, making sure it is well spread out.

4 Bake in the oven for 25–30 minutes until slightly toasted and well dried out.

5 Leave to cool before storing in labelled sandwich bags.

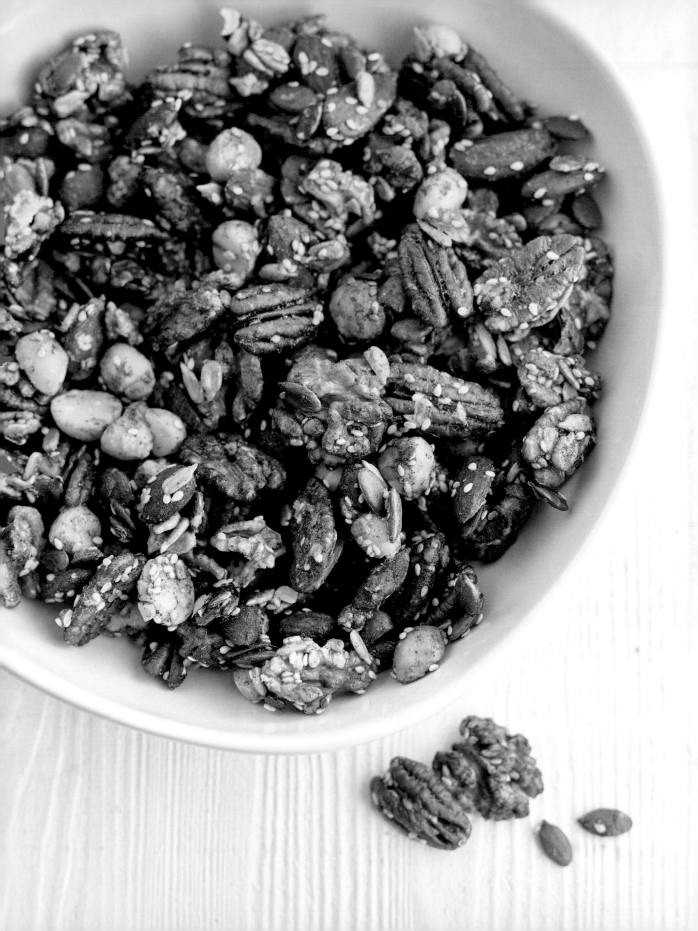

CARROT, WALNUT AND SPELT LOAF

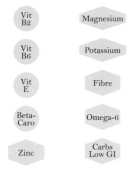

Vit B2 · Magnesium

Vit B6 · Potassium

Vit E · Fibre

Beta-Caro · Omega-6

Zinc · Carbs Low GI

Carrots are naturally sweet, and therefore so is this bread, which is the perfect snack to have in between meals. A couple of slices of this will see you through to dinnertime while ensuring you are getting lots of fibre, goodness from the seeds and nuts, and a little sugar lift from the sweetness in the carrots and honey.

PREP TIME 15 MINUTES • COOK TIME 45 MINUTES • MAKES 1 LOAF

75ml rapeseed oil, plus extra for greasing
250g spelt flour
100g walnuts
1 tsp caraway seeds
½ tsp mixed spice
2 heaped tsp baking powder
75ml almond milk
100g carrot, peeled and grated
4 tbsp runny honey
pinch of salt
75g sunflower seeds

1 Preheat the oven to 180°C (fan 160°C) and grease a 750g non-stick loaf tin.

2 Place the flour, walnuts and caraway seeds in a food processor, and pulse for 2–3 minutes to form a rough powder. Add the remaining ingredients, except the sunflower seeds, and blend until the mixture is well combined. Fold in half the sunflower seeds.

3 Tip into the prepared tin and sprinkle with the remaining sunflower seeds. Bake for 45 minutes until the top is golden brown and a skewer inserted into the centre of the bread comes out clean.

4 Remove the loaf from the tin and leave to cool on a wire rack before storing in an airtight container for up to 1 week.

PARMESAN SEEDED CRISPBREADS

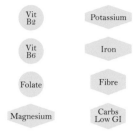

Vit B2
Potassium
Vit B6
Iron
Folate
Fibre
Magnesium
Carbs Low GI

The ultimate storecupboard snack. I love these with my Avocado and Cumin Dip (page 180), dipped into Sumac and Tahini Hummus (page 181), layered with a chunk of cheese and some pickle, or simply on their own. Make a batch for whenever you need a quick snack. (See the photograph on pages 182–83).

PREP TIME 10 MINUTES • COOK TIME 15–20 MINUTES • MAKES 12–14

225g buckwheat flour
225g wholemeal flour
75g sunflower seeds
75g pumpkin seeds
2 tbsp milled flaxseed
2 tbsp sesame seeds
75g pinhead or rolled oats
2 tbsp chia seeds
1 tsp salt
150ml extra virgin rapeseed
   or olive oil

FOR THE TOPPING
50g Parmesan cheese,
   finely grated
2 tbsp poppy seeds

1 Preheat the oven to 200°C (fan 180°C) and cut 2 pieces of parchment the same size as a large flat baking tray.

2 Mix all the dry ingredients in a bowl, then make a well in the centre and add the oil, followed by 120ml cold water. Mix with your fingertips to form a dough. Slowly add up to a further 120ml cold water until the dough is firm but not sticky – you may not need all the water. Form the dough into a ball.

3 Place the ball onto one piece of parchment and lay the second piece on top. Using the heel of your hand, flatten the dough before using a rolling pin to roll it out to the same size as your baking tray. It should be about ½cm thick.

4 Lift the parchment with the rolled dough onto the baking tray, remove the top sheet of parchment and sprinkle over the Parmesan and poppy seeds. Bake for 15–20 minutes until the dough goes hard and golden brown. Turn the tray around halfway through cooking to ensure even cooking.

5 Once cooked, remove the tray from the oven and peel off the parchment from underneath the crispbread. Use a large sharp knife – or snap the crispbread with your hands for a more rustic effect – into your desired shapes and sizes. I like random shapes, some big and some small. Leave to cool on a wire rack before storing in an airtight container or sandwich bags for up to 1 week.

AVOCADO AND CUMIN DIP

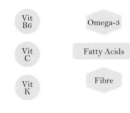

This dip is multi-functional – it's great on its own, served with crispy snacks and crudités, but it will also work in the Ultimate Chicken and Avocado Burger (see page 130), spooned into Blackened Fish with Guacamole and Black-eyed Bean Tacos (see page 104), or with anything that needs a little greenery and something moist. (See the photograph on page 183.)

PREP TIME 10 MINUTES • MAKES 4 PORTIONS

1 large ripe avocado
1 tsp ground cumin, plus extra to serve
15g fresh coriander leaves, finely chopped
zest and juice of 2 limes
2–3 tbsp extra virgin rapeseed oil, olive oil or avocado oil, plus extra to serve
salt and freshly ground black pepper

1 Cut the avocado in half and remove the stone. Scoop the flesh into a food processor along with all the other ingredients. Blend until completely smooth and season with a little salt and pepper.

2 Pour into a small airtight container and cover with a sheet of cling film to prevent it oxidising before placing on the lid, ready to eat as and when you wish. The dip with keep for 2–3 days in the fridge if stored correctly.

3 If serving in a bowl, sprinkle the top with a little more cumin and a drizzle of oil before serving.

BEETROOT AND HAZELNUT DIP

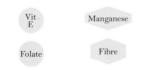

The hazelnuts in this vibrant dip not only add a natural creaminess but also a lovely dose of vitamin E, great for healthy skin and reducing the risk of developing stretch marks. (See the photograph on page 182.)

PREP TIME 10 MINUTES • MAKES 1 LARGE TUB

300g cooked, unpickled beetroot
100g hazelnuts, skins on, toasted
zest of 1 large orange
1 tsp ground cumin
2 tbsp natural yogurt
3 tbsp extra virgin rapeseed, olive oil or flaxseed oil
salt and freshly ground black pepper

Blitz all the ingredients in a large blender or food processor until smooth. Season with salt and pepper, and serve, or place in a sealed airtight container and eat as and when you wish. This dip will keep for 2–3 days in the fridge.

SUMAC AND TAHINI HUMMUS

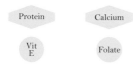

Tahini is the sesame seed paste that gives hummus its distinctive flavour. I like to use a lot of it here. Not only does it enhance the taste, but it also contains vitamin E, calcium and folate. Vitamin E is great for supple skin, helping prevent stretch marks. Calcium is needed for healthy bones and folate will help with fatigue. (See the photograph on page 183.)

PREP TiME 10 MINUTES • MAKES 1 LARGE TUB

1 x 400g tin chickpeas,
   rinsed and drained
1–2 garlic cloves, peeled
   and grated
2 tbsp tahini paste
zest and juice of 1 lemon
6 tbsp extra virgin rapeseed
   or olive oil, plus
   extra to drizzle
3 tsp sumac, plus extra
   to sprinkle
pinch of ground cumin
salt

1 Place all the ingredients with a pinch of salt in a blender and blitz to form a smooth paste. This will take about 3 minutes. Once blended, taste for seasoning; you may feel it needs a little more lemon. If you think it should be a little looser, add a little more oil and blend again.

2 Transfer the hummus to an airtight container, sprinkle with a little more sumac and a drizzle of oil, and store in the fridge until you fancy a snack – it will keep for 2–3 days.

NUT BUTTER

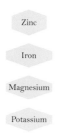

Nut butters are extremely easy to make. You can, of course, buy them in supermarkets or health-food shops, but I find that I quite regularly have half a bag of nuts in my cupboard and as they tend to go off quite quickly, I make them into nut butter, which I can then spread on toast or breakfast loaf in the morning, or stir through my porridge. Nut butters are also great added to homemade pesto and stirred through pasta.

Nuts are a key part of our diets, especially while pregnant, as they are rich in essential fats and nutrients.

PREP TIME 10 MINUTES • MAKES 300G

300g raw almonds, cashews,
   hazelnuts or Brazil nuts
1 tbsp runny honey

Blend the nuts in a food processor for 2 minutes, then scrape down the sides and add the honey. Blend in 2-minute bursts until completely smooth. This will take about 10 minutes. Store in an airtight container in the fridge and use within 3–4 days.

BEETROOT AND
HAZELENUT DIP
(PAGE 180)

PARMESAN SEEDED
CRISPBREAD
(PAGE 179)

AVOCADO AND
CUMIN DIP
(PAGE 180)

SUMAC AND
TAHINI HUMMUS
(PAGE 181)

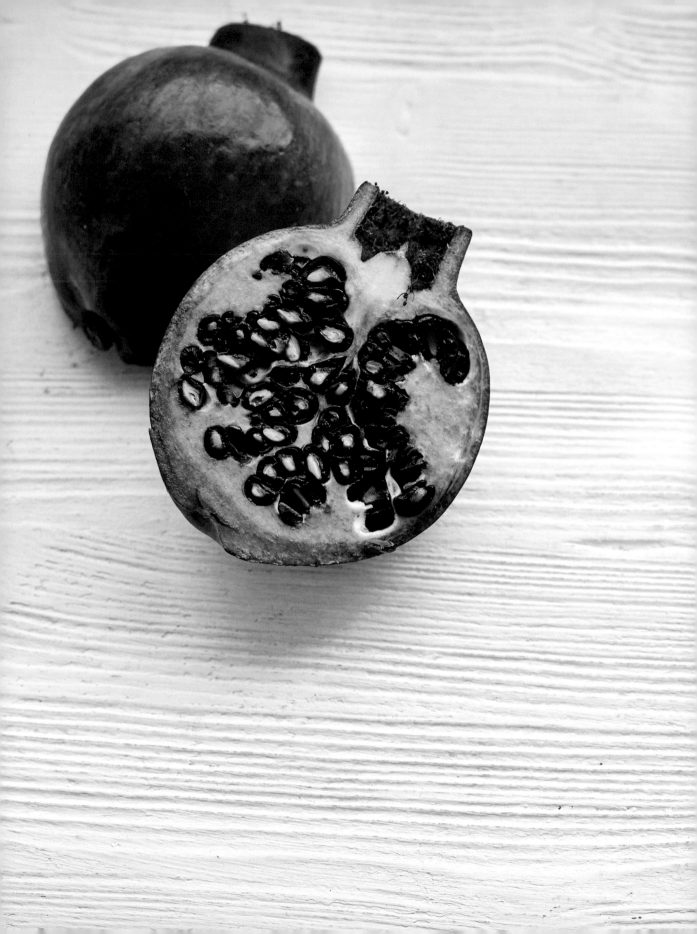

SWEET TREATS

Although this is a healthy pregnancy cookbook, I had to include a few delicious sweet treats for you! Being pregnant isn't an easy job, and us girls have to put up with a lot: our ever-changing shape, aching feet and back, nausea, bloating, indigestion – you get the gist! It's therefore my job to help you to create a few delicious indulgences that will not only satisfy a craving for something sweet, but also add nutrients and vitamins to your diet without you even knowing it.

Desserts and yummy sweet treats are fine for us to eat in moderation, and should be enjoyed whenever you feel you need them. Bake a batch of healthy Date and Almond Flapjacks (page 195) once a week and share them with work colleagues or family. Try my Almond, Banana and Strawberry Milk Lollies (page 188) when the sun is shining, and the Banana, Date and Coconut Energy Truffles (page 192) are perfect for packing into your bag when you're out and about.

These are desserts the whole family can enjoy, created with health and nutrition for you and your baby at the forefront of my mind so that you can sit back, relax and enjoy your treat without feeling guilty. For more information on sugar and sugar substitutes, see page 19.

Although the recipes in this section are all very quick and easy to prepare, I also appreciate that sometimes you just need something NOW! Here are a few (healthy) instant sweet snacks to fill the gap:

* Sliced apple drizzled with runny honey and scattered with toasted flaked almonds.

* Pineapple chunks tossed in lime juice and torn fresh mint leaves.

* Ripe pear or fig with a slice of salty Parmesan cheese.

* Fresh berries (blueberries, strawberries or raspberries) and torn fresh mint leaves, drizzled with agave or runny honey.

* A handful of mixed dried fruits and nuts.

* A square or two of dark chocolate.

ALMOND, BANANA AND STRAWBERRY MILK LOLLIES

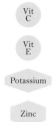

Vit C

Vit E

Potassium

Zinc

Who says lollies are just for kiddies? I am currently 34 weeks pregnant and particularly partial to something ice-cold. I just can't seem to quench my constant thirst, so lollies are a great treat when a glass of sparkling water or iced tea just won't cut it, especially on a hot day.

Bananas give the lollies their thick and creamy texture, and also work as a natural sweetener. Strawberries are a great source of vitamin C, essential in the preconception stage and throughout pregnancy to maintain a healthy mum and eventually baby.

PREP TIME 15 MINUTES • FREEZE TIME 3 HOURS • MAKES 12

100g strawberries
600ml almond milk
3 very ripe large bananas
3 tbsp runny honey

12 lolly moulds or small disposable cups
12 wooden lolly sticks

1 Hull and finely chop the strawberries before placing them in a small saucepan with a tablespoon of cold water. Simmer over a low heat until the strawberries start to break down slightly, stirring all the time. Once the strawberries resemble a chunky compote, after about 8–10 minutes, turn off the heat and allow to cool completely in the fridge.

2 Blend together the almond milk, bananas and honey until completely smooth. Pour the mixture into the lolly moulds and place in the freezer for 30 minutes. After this time, remove the lolly moulds from the freezer and drop 2–3 teaspoons of the cooled strawberry compote into the partially frozen lolly mixture. Use the lolly stick to ripple the strawberry through the almond milk mixture. Place the sticks in the middle of the lolly moulds and return to the freezer for about 2½ hours. Once frozen they are ready to eat.

3 The lollies will last for up to 1 month in the freezer. If you find you are not eating your lollies, you can use them in your morning smoothie.

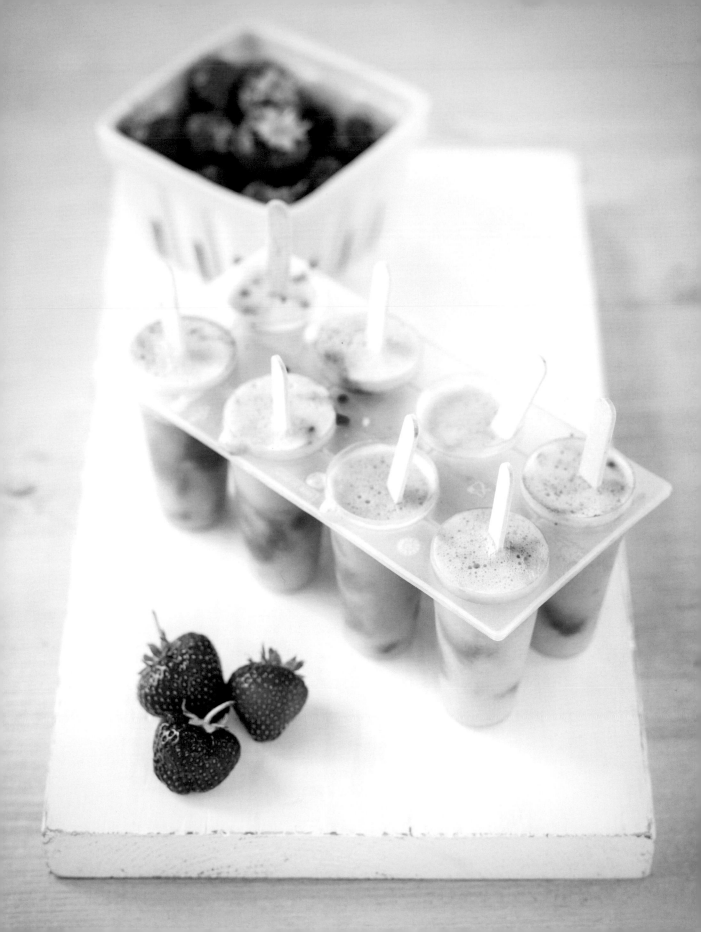

GOOEY CHOCOLATE, PRUNE AND SWEET POTATO SQUARES

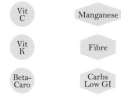

Vit C

Vit K

Beta-Caro

Manganese

Fibre

Carbs Low GI

You may think this sounds crazy, but trust me. The sweet potato in this recipe keeps the cake so moist that it completely removes the need for butter, and it is so naturally sweet that very little added sweetness is required to make this cake perfectly balanced and a real treat for those of us with a sweet tooth.

Prunes are naturally sticky and sweet, as well as containing lots of fibre, which will help to keep your digestive system regular. Sweet potatoes are a fantastic source of beta-carotene, which in the third trimester is important for your baby's eye development.

PREP TIME 10 MINUTES • COOK TIME 50 MINUTES • MAKES 8–10 SLICES OR 12–16 SMALLER SQUARES

2 tbsp coconut oil, plus extra for greasing
2 large sweet potatoes (about 600g), or you can also use butternut squash
150g pitted prunes
5 tbsp runny honey
2 tsp vanilla bean paste or vanilla extract
150g buckwheat, rye or wholewheat flour
100g cocoa powder, plus extra to sprinkle
200g ground almonds
1 tsp baking powder

1 Preheat the oven to 200°C (fan 180°C) and grease and line a 20cm square brownie tin with parchment.

2 Bake the whole sweet potatoes in the oven for 30 minutes until tender. You can also do this in the microwave on full power for 8–10 minutes if you are in a rush. Once the sweet potatoes are cooked and completely tender, remove them from the oven and cut them in half lengthways. Scoop out the filling using a large spoon. You can do this by holding each half in a clean tea towel if they are hot, or alternatively just wait until they are cool enough to handle.

3 Place the sweet potato flesh in a food processor, along with the prunes, coconut oil, honey and vanilla, and blend until completely smooth. Add the flour, cocoa powder, ground almonds and baking powder, and blend again. Pour the mixture into the prepared tin and bake for 20–25 minutes. Once the top is set and the middle is still slightly squidgy, it is ready.

4 Leave to cool before sprinkling with a little more cocoa powder. Portion and serve with fresh berries and Greek yogurt as a dessert. Alternatively, cut into mini squares and serve as you would a brownie, with a nice hot drink.

PEANUT BUTTER, BANANA AND OATMEAL COOKIES

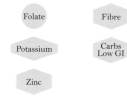

Folate

Potassium

Zinc

Fibre

Carbs
Low GI

These cookies are not only a nice treat but also a good source of fibre and folate, which is greatly needed throughout your pregnancy. I often make the dough and keep a little batch in the freezer, already portioned, so I can bake a fresh batch of cookies whenever guests pop in.

They are not overly sweet like many cookies, so you can have a few in your handbag for those days when you have to commute and might need a quick fix to keep nausea at bay, or when hunger really strikes during the third trimester.

PREP TIME 10 MINUTES • COOK TIME 13–16 MINUTES • MAKES 16

2 large over-ripe bananas
4 tbsp crunchy peanut
    butter, unsweetened
2 tbsp almond milk or semi-
    skimmed cows' milk
3 tbsp runny honey
4 dates, chopped
1 tbsp chocolate-hazelnut
    spread
8 tbsp rolled porridge oats
1 tsp ground cinnamon
3 tbsp bran or wholemeal
    flour

1 Preheat the oven to 200°C (fan 180°C) and line a large baking tray with parchment.

2 In a large bowl, mash the bananas with a fork until smooth. Add the peanut butter, milk, honey, dates and chocolate-hazelnut spread, and mix well. Now add the dry ingredients and stir until well combined.

3 Roll spoonfuls of dough in your hands and place them on the prepared baking tray, then flatten slightly into cookie shapes. Bake in the oven for 13–16 minutes until golden and still slightly squidgy. Remove from the oven and leave the cookies to cool on a wire rack before storing in an airtight container for up to 1 week.

4 You can also freeze the shaped cookie dough for warm cookies straight from the oven whenever you feel the need. Simply bake them from frozen in a 200°C (fan 180°C) oven for 16–18 minutes.

BANANA, DATE AND COCONUT ENERGY TRUFFLES

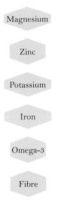

Magnesium

Zinc

Potassium

Iron

Omega-3

Fibre

These little energy bites are popping up in all the health-food shops at the moment. They are so easy to make at home, where you can add whatever flavours and ingredients you like, making them bespoke to you and your tastes throughout your pregnancy.

I made these while in my first trimester as I was totally exhausted and needed the occasional energy boost but didn't want to rely on sugary biscuits and chocolate bars to fix my cravings. They offer a great injection of energy when it comes to elevenses, especially when paired with a crunchy apple or a handful of nuts to boost your intake of protein, fibre and much-needed minerals for you and your growing baby.

PREP TIME 15 MINUTES • MAKES 30

250g whole almonds
100g pecan nuts
200g pitted dates
2 over-ripe bananas
2 tsp chia seeds
2 tsp flaxseeds
2 tsp cocoa powder
1 tsp ground cinnamon

FOR THE COATING
100g desiccated coconut

1 Put the almonds and pecans into a food processor and blend for 3–4 minutes until they turn to powder. Add the remaining ingredients and blend again to form a paste.

2 Mould the paste into 30 small balls. I find this easier if I wet my hands first, to stop the mixture sticking too much. Roll each ball in the desiccated coconut. Place the balls on a tray, cover well with cling film and place in the freezer. Once the balls are hard, you can transfer them from the tray into freezer bags. Label the bags with the contents and the date made. They will keep in the freezer for up to 1 month.

3 They are delicious served at room temperature or when just starting to defrost.

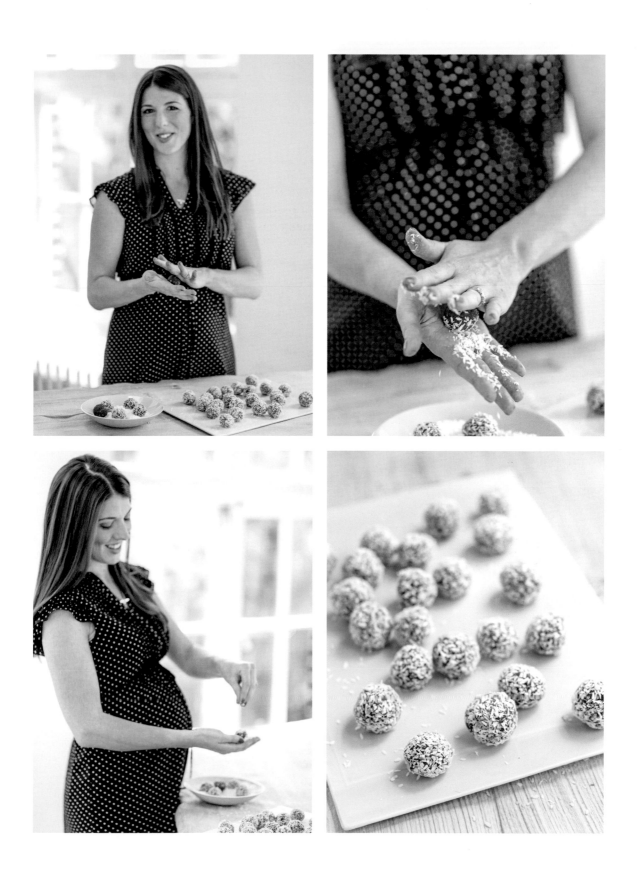

COCOA AND AVOCADO MOUSSE CAKE

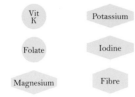

Vit K

Potassium

Folate

Iodine

Magnesium

Fibre

Because avocados have such a rich and silky texture that remains moist once cooked, they make a fabulous addition to baking. Not only that, but because of their high healthy fat content, they can actually replace butter in many recipes. I love making this cake and watching people's reactions when I tell them it's made with avocados. They look at me like I'm crazy.

Avocados are a lovely source of fibre, vitamin K and folate, among other good things, and should be introduced into our diets while pregnant as much as possible. They may also help to relieve constipation in some ladies, due to the high amounts of essential fatty acids they contain, which help to keep the digestive system lubricated.

PREP TIME 15 MINUTES • COOK TIME 35–40 MINUTES • SERVES 8

avocado or olive oil,
   for greasing
200g good quality raw
   or 70–80 per cent dark
   chocolate, broken
   into pieces
120g runny honey
175g ground almonds
2 tsp baking powder
1 large ripe avocado
3 free-range eggs,
   separated

1 Preheat the oven to 180°C (fan 160°C) and grease a 20cm loose-bottomed cake tin before lining it with parchment.

2 Put the chocolate and honey in a heatproof bowl set over a pan of simmering water. Don't allow the water to boil or let the bottom of the bowl touch the simmering water. Stir until all the chocolate has melted. Remove from the heat and leave to cool – you want it to be cool enough that it doesn't start to cook the eggs when you add them.

3 Once the chocolate has cooled, add the almonds and baking powder and gently fold them into the melted chocolate.

4 Blend the avocado with the 3 egg yolks and fold into the chocolate mixture. Whisk the 3 egg whites to firm peaks and fold them in too, carefully ensuring everything is well combined.

4 Pour the mixture into the prepared cake tin and bake in the oven for 35–40 minutes. Check to make sure the cake is cooked by inserting a skewer into the centre; if the skewer comes out clean, the cake is cooked. Remove the cake from the oven and leave to cool slightly before serving with a little soured cream and a dusting of cocoa powder. You can store the cake in an airtight container, out of the fridge, for 2–3 days.

DATE AND ALMOND FLAPJACKS

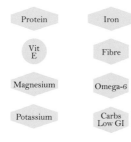

Protein
Vit E
Magnesium
Potassium
Iron
Fibre
Omega-6
Carbs Low GI

I have to admit that I am slightly addicted to these flapjacks! I never had a sweet tooth before falling pregnant but now, especially as I move further into the third trimester, I find myself craving sweet things. I find a good trick is to cut these flapjacks a little smaller than you might usually, meaning you eat a little less and don't have to feel bad about your sugar fix. I have added lots of fruit and nuts to make the flapjacks rich in fibre, potassium and magnesium. Almonds especially provide a very good source of magnesium, which can help to reduce anxiety during pregnancy, help your muscles relax, and reduce stress.

PREP TIME 10 MINUTES • COOK TIME 16–20 MINUTES • MAKES 16

8 tbsp coconut oil, melted, plus extra for greasing
225g pitted dates
150g almonds
150g pecans
2 tsp ground ginger
1 tsp ground nutmeg
400g rolled porridge oats
8 tbsp maple syrup
6 tbsp mixed seeds

1 Preheat the oven to 200°C (fan 180°C) and grease a 20cm square brownie tin with a little coconut oil.

2 Put the dates, almonds, pecans, ginger and nutmeg in a food processor and blitz to a rough paste. Add the oats, maple syrup and melted coconut oil, and blend again for 30 seconds.

3 Transfer the flapjack mixture to the prepared tin and pack it down firmly, making sure the surface is even. Now sprinkle over the mixed seeds and press down again. Bake for 16–20 minutes until slightly golden around the edges. Remove the tray from the oven and, using a sharp knife, cut the flapjacks into squares while still warm in the tin. Leave to cool in the tin before storing in an airtight container for up to 1 week.

FROZEN GREEK YOGURT AND POMEGRANATE CUBES

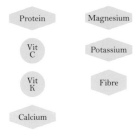

These look so pretty and are extremely satisfying to eat, especially when it's hot. You can literally pop one or two out of your ice-cube tray whenever you like, getting a good kick of calcium, which is great for your baby's growing and hardening bones and teeth, while refreshing and cleansing your palate at the same time. I've also yet to find kids who don't love these, so they are great to have in the freezer on a warm day if you have little ones already or are expecting family or friends to pop round with their brood.

Pomegranates not only look beautiful and taste divine, but they are rich in vitamins C and K, both important throughout your pregnancy and for a healthy immune system.

PREP TIME 10 MINUTES • MAKES 2 TRAYS (24 CUBES)

juice of 1 lemon
4–5 tbsp sugar, agave
  or Xylitol
500g 2 per cent fat
  Greek yogurt
200g pomegranate seeds

1 Mix the lemon juice with the sugar in a small saucepan and heat very gently until the sugar has dissolved. Add this to the yogurt and stir through the pomegranate seeds. Spoon or pour the mixture into ice-cube trays and freeze for 2–3 hours until they have set hard. Once frozen, cover the trays with cling film until ready to eat.

2 You can also drop these into a smoothie in the morning if you find you have made too many.

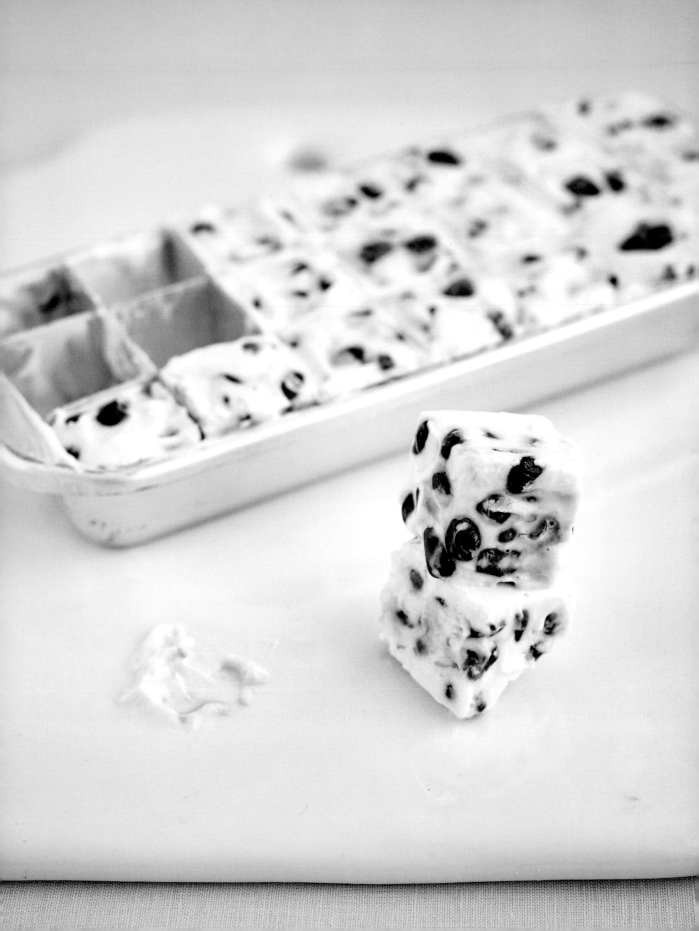

GO 'NUTTY' FOR BANANA BREAD

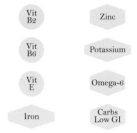

Vit B2
Vit B6
Vit E
Iron
Zinc
Potassium
Omega-6
Carbs Low GI

Banana bread is something very special indeed. I've been perfecting this recipe during my pregnancy and I think I finally have it! I've tried to add as much goodness as I possibly can while keeping the sugar levels low. It is a very dense loaf and can be enjoyed as an energy boost in bite-sized pieces or simply sliced and served with a cup of tea whenever you fancy something wholesome and delicious.

This recipe contains lots of delicious seeds and nuts, which are brilliant sources of vitamins B and E, iron and zinc, all of which are essential to promote fertility and to support a growing baby. My husband is also a big fan, so everyone's happy.

PREP TIME 15 MINUTES • COOK TIME 1¼–1½ HOURS • MAKES 1 LOAF

2 tbsp rapeseed oil, plus extra for greasing
3 large ripe bananas
12 pitted organic dates
100g pecan nuts
250g buckwheat, wholemeal or brown rice flour
75g ground almonds
2 tsp baking powder
1 tsp ground cinnamon
1 tsp ground mixed spice
2 free-range eggs
120ml almond milk or semi-skimmed cows' milk
3 tbsp runny honey

FOR THE TOP
2 tbsp mixed pumpkin seeds, sunflower seeds and flaked almonds

1 Preheat the oven to 180°C (fan 160°C) and grease and line a 750g loaf tin with parchment.

2 Place the bananas, dates and pecans in a food processor and blend until you have a rough-textured paste. Add the flour, ground almonds, baking powder, cinnamon and mixed spice, and blend until smooth. Crack in the eggs, one at a time, while blending, before adding the milk, oil and honey. Blend again.

3 Pour the mixture into the prepared loaf tin and sprinkle generously with the seeds and flaked almonds. Bake in the oven for 1¼–1½ hours. Check the loaf is cooked by inserting a skewer into the centre; if it comes out clean, the banana bread is cooked. Leave to cool for at least 20 minutes before serving with a cuppa. Go on… you deserve it!

STRAWBERRY, BASIL
AND COCONUT ICE

Vit C

Vit E

Potassium

You can make this recipe with many different ingredients, but I love this combination. I'm usually the person wearing three layers while my husband walks round in a T-shirt, but as my bump grows I find that I am getting really hot and bothered with only seven weeks to go. I love walking to the freezer and scooping out a few tablespoons of this coconut ice. It really cools me down and also gives me a little fix when I am having a sweetie craving. It contains lots of vitamin C, and as the strawberries are raw, they keep hold of their nutrients and vitamins, meaning you and baby really benefit from them.

PREP TIME 10 MINUTES • FREEZING TIME 4–6 HOURS • MAKES 1.25 LITRES

400g frozen strawberries
60ml agave nectar
12 fresh basil leaves
800ml coconut milk

1 Blitz all the ingredients in a blender until smooth. Pour into an airtight container and place in the freezer. Stir the mixture every 20–30 minutes, using a fork to break up the ice crystals. It is ready to serve when it is frozen but still contains small, broken ice crystals. It will take around 4–6 hours to freeze completely.

2 To serve, spoon over some fresh fruit or, better still, the pulp of a passion fruit.

3 This granita or frozen ice will keep in the freezer for up to 1 month. You may need to break up the ice crystals every time you want to eat it, which is easily done using a fork.

GINGER, GOJI BERRY AND PISTACHIO COCOA SNAPS

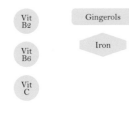

Vit B2

Vit B6

Vit C

Gingerols

Iron

There is no better treat than one that can be made in advance and left to look after itself in the fridge. There is no cooking involved in this recipe; it can simply be prepared and left to set. This recipe always reminds me of my mum, as she would serve chocolate-covered ginger with coffee after a meal, which as a kid I hated but of course now have become rather fond of. There is something very 'grown-up' about enjoying the taste of bitter rich dark chocolate and hot heady ginger with a cup of (now decaffeinated) strong black coffee.

PREP TIME 20 MINUTES, PLUS 2 HOURS SETTING TIME
• MAKES 12–15 LARGE SHARDS

200g good quality 80 per cent dark chocolate
2 tbsp coconut oil
½ tsp ground ginger
pinch of salt
3 tbsp stem ginger syrup or runny honey
3 tbsp goji berries or chopped dried figs (try to buy the soft, unsulphured variety)
1 tbsp stem ginger, finely chopped
1 tbsp chia seeds
3 tbsp peeled pistachio nuts
3 tbsp blanched almonds

1 Line a large flat baking tray with a sheet of parchment.

2 Half-fill a small saucepan with water, bring to the boil, then turn the heat down low. Place the chocolate and coconut oil in a heatproof bowl that fits directly over but not touching the simmering water and allow the chocolate to melt, stirring regularly. Once melted, leave to cool to body temperature.

3 Once you can dip your little finger into the chocolate without it feeling either hot or cold, it's perfect. Add the ground ginger, salt and stem ginger syrup or honey, and stir well. Pour the melted chocolate onto the prepared baking tray. Mix the goji berries, stem ginger, chia seeds and nuts together before scattering over the top of the melted chocolate.

4 Place the tray in the fridge for 2 hours to set. Once set, break the sheet into shards and store in an airtight container in the fridge, ready to serve as and when fancied (or needed).

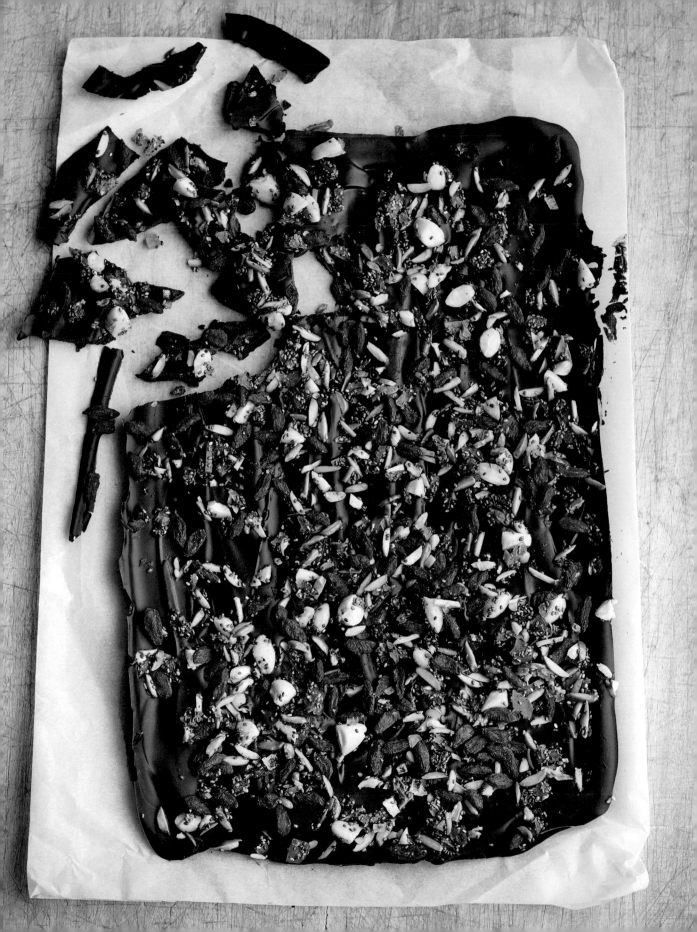

NAKED MANGO
AND RASPBERRY TREATS

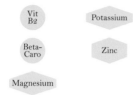

Vit B2

Potassium

Beta-Caro

Zinc

Magnesium

I love dried mango and always have a packet or two in my cupboard at home, so I set about creating a recipe to incorporate this tasty treat into something a bit more substantial which would really give me a lift in the middle of the day as my sugar levels started to crash.

Dried mango is a great source of beta-carotene, which helps prevent eye defects in growing baby. It can also reduce the risk of pre-eclampsia in mum.

PREP TIME 10 MINUTES • SETTING TIME 1 HOUR • MAKES 12

80g coconut oil, melted
125g whole blanched almonds
125g desiccated coconut
250g soft, unsulphured dried mango
3 tbsp runny honey
100g freeze-dried raspberries, ground to a powder

1 Grease a 500g loaf tin with a little coconut oil and line it with a thin strip of greaseproof paper. Ensure the strip hangs over both ends of the tin. This will create a little handle to help remove your treat once it is set.

2 Blitz the almonds to a fine powder in a food processor. Add the desiccated coconut, mango and honey, and blend again for 3–4 minutes until you have a smooth paste. Add the coconut oil and blend for another minute or so.

3 Spoon the mixture into the prepared tin. Compact it well using the back of a spoon and even out the surface. Sprinkle with the freeze-dried raspberries before transferring the tin to the fridge for 1 hour to set. Once set, remove from the fridge and, using the handles, remove your treat from the tin.

4 Portion the slab into 12 pieces. These can now be wrapped in greaseproof paper and stored in the fridge, ready to be eaten as a tasty snack. Alternatively, they can be portioned into bags and kept in the freezer for up to 1 month. Remove from the freezer 2–3 hours before eating.

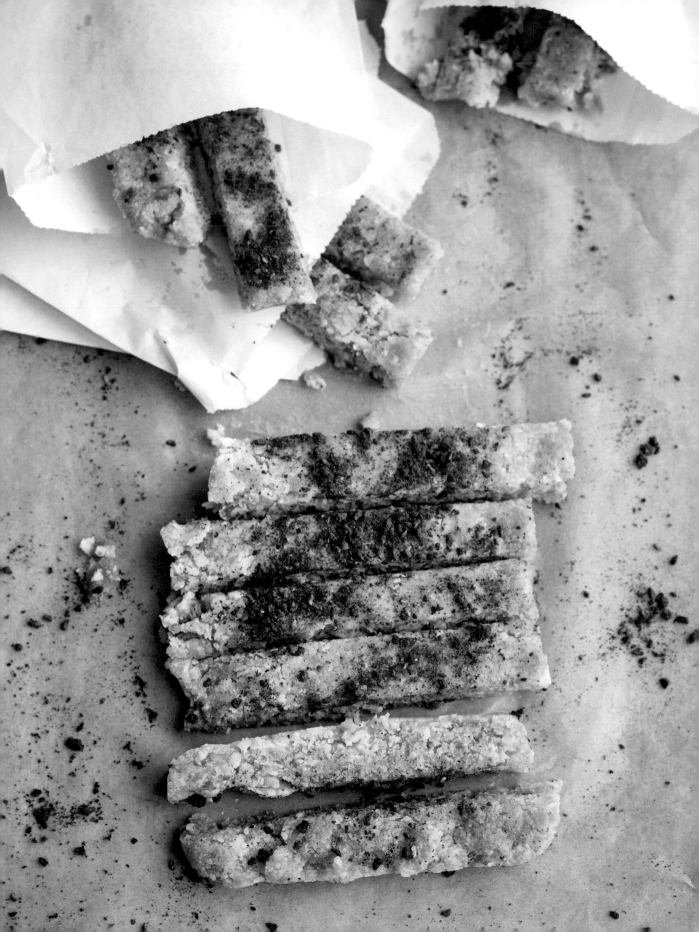

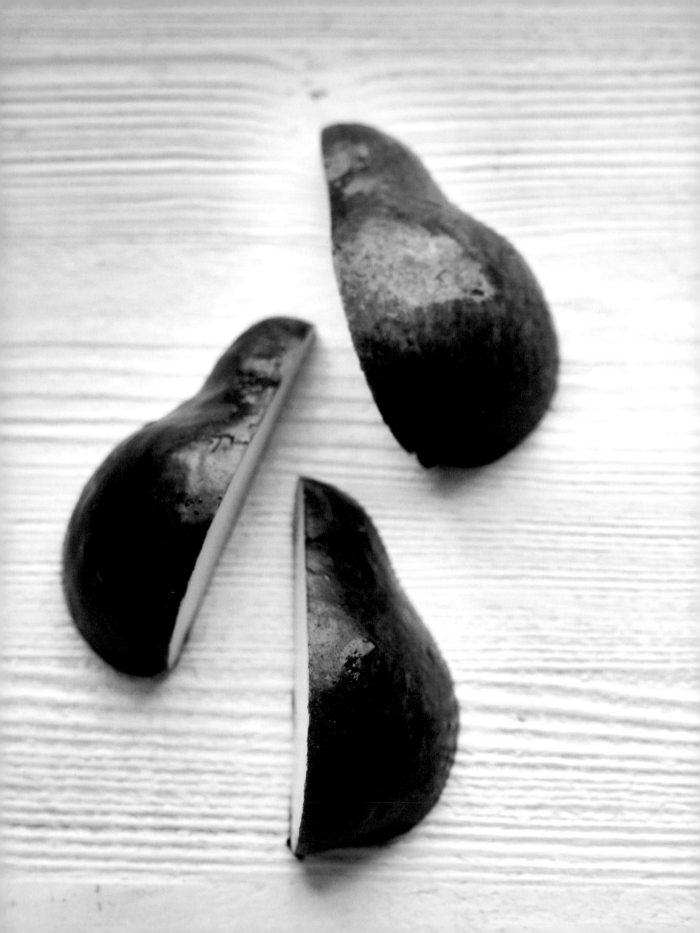

JUICES, SMOOTHIES, TEAS AND WARMING DRINKS

A smoothie or juice is by no means a substitute for a meal, but it is an ideal way of consuming extra nutrients. I have a juice most mornings, which I make in my juicer. There are lots of different types of juicers on the market; mine is a centrifugal one, but you could also use a slow-grind juicer for these recipes, although they will take a little longer to make.

The ingredients I choose to juice depend on how I am feeling and which vegetables and fruits I feel I need an 'injection' of. If you are going to add citrus juice to your juices, you will need to squeeze the juice separately, as you can't juice whole oranges and lemons. You can juice whole limes, but I wouldn't recommend it as the pith is bitter and may taint the flavour of your juice. If the recipe calls for coconut water, simply add this through the top of the juicer after all the other ingredients, as it will help to extract every last drop of juice remaining in the juicer, meaning you won't miss out on a single drop of goodness! Juices need to be consumed as soon as you have prepared them, as they will oxidise and separate if left for too long, especially if they contain apple or pear.

Smoothies are a great way of using up leftovers in the fridge or fruit bowl and they have the added benefit of extra fibre, which juices are missing, making them more filling. I often make a smoothie for elevenses or if I am leaving the house in a rush and need a quick something to line my stomach. A smoothie can be a healthy fill-in if you are a little short of time or need to load up on the extra calories you will need in your third trimester or when breastfeeding. A smoothie should be made and consumed the same day. It doesn't keep well in the fridge as it also tends to split and oxidise, especially if it contains banana. If you would like to include some extra calcium in your diet, add a couple of tablespoons of natural yogurt to your smoothie, or make it with cows' milk. To make a smoothie is easy: simply place all the ingredients in a blender and blitz until silky smooth. Don't peel or remove anything, unless it really is totally indigestible – like citrus peel, banana peel or pineapple skin, stones and pips – and do make sure you give anything you blend a really good wash beforehand.

I have also chosen to include a few comforting and warming drinks in this chapter. These are particularly good in the evening for when you're enjoying a bit of down time or if you are in need of 'a hug in a mug'. As well as being nutritionally beneficial, they will also serve as a substitute for your usual daily dose of hot drinks such as tea or coffee which should be consumed in moderation in pregnancy or when trying to conceive.

These recipes are my own personal favourites, but play around with ingredients to make your own delicious drinks. All the recipes in this chapter make enough for 1 serving – apart from my Mulled Apple, Cinnamon and Anise drink (page 213), which makes a great non-alcoholic alternative to mulled wine or cider during the party season!

JUICES

Juices are quick to make and they are a great way of getting an instant hit of nutrients. You do need a special juicer but there are some good fairly cheap ones available now. These are some of my favourite combinations – see page 206 for some juicing tips.

VISUALLY PERFECT

Vit C
Beta-Caro
Gingerols

Great for baby's eye development.

4 carrots
7cm piece fresh ginger, peeled
10 fresh mint leaves
juice of 1 lemon
juice of 2 oranges

REHYDRATER

Vit C
Iron
Folate

A great way to quench your thirst, thanks to the coconut water, with the added benefit of many essential vitamins and minerals.

2 handfuls of baby leaf spinach
½ cucumber
3 oranges
250ml coconut water

PICK-ME-UP

Vit C
Gingerols

The fennel and ginger in this juice may help give you a little relief from morning sickness.

2 green apples
2 pears
5cm piece fresh ginger, peeled
10 fresh mint leaves
½ fennel bulb

OESTROGEN BOOST

Vit C
Vit K
Iron
Omega-3
Fibre

High in iron and essential vitamins for a stronger immune system.

2 handfuls of kale
handful of baby leaf spinach
2 celery sticks
¼ fennel bulb
1 pear
1 green apple
juice of 1 lemon

FOLATE LIFT

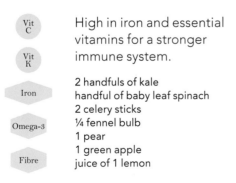

Vit C
Iron
Folate

Perfect for a folate or iron deficiency.

2 celery sticks
1 large beetroot
2 apples
2 handfuls of baby leaf spinach or kale
75g broccoli florets
juice of 1 lemon
juice of 1 orange

SMOOTHIES

Smoothies contain more fibre than juices so are great for staving off hunger between mealtimes or if you're in a hurry and need a quick fix. They are also a great way of getting in extra nutrients. Play around with your favourite ingredients – see page 206 for some smoothie-making tips.

GLOWING NUTTY: ALMOND AND BANANA

The sugar content will help lift energy levels, while vitamin E will help towards keeping your skin supple, reducing the likelihood of stretch marks.

200ml semi-skimmed milk or unsweetened almond milk
1 tbsp cocoa powder
100g blanched raw almonds
1 large ripe banana, peeled
1 tbsp manuka honey

THE REFRESHER: MELON, MINT AND KIWI

Folate
Iron
Fibre

The perfect drink to quench your thirst and inject a few essential vitamins to boost your immune system.

½ cucumber
100g honeydew melon, frozen
1 handful seedless white grapes
1 kiwi fruit
handful of baby leaf spinach
10 fresh mint leaves
juice of 1 lemon
handful of ice
you may need a dash of water of coconut water to loosen your smoothie a little

GREEN OMEGA: AVOCADO AND BANANA

High in omega-3 and fatty acids, essential for both mum and growing baby.

1 avocado, stone removed and peeled
2 handfuls of baby leaf spinach
1 banana, peeled
1 green apple
1 tbsp milled flaxseed
200ml coconut water

BREAKFAST ON THE GO: BLUEBERRIES, PRUNES AND OATS

Potassium
Magnesium
Zinc
Fibre

Filling and substantial, with enough calories to get you through the morning.

200ml almond milk
3 tbsp frozen blueberries
3 pitted prunes
1 large ripe banana, peeled
2 tbsp almond butter
1 tbsp rolled porridge oats
1 tbsp milled flaxseed

HUNGER FIX: PEANUT AND BANANA

Protein
Potassium
Iron
Folate
Omega-3
Choline

The perfect snack to keep you going until lunchtime.

200ml unsweetened almond milk
2 tsp cocoa powder
2 tbsp peanut butter
handful of baby leaf spinach
1 frozen peeled and chopped banana
handful of ice
1 tbsp milled flaxseed

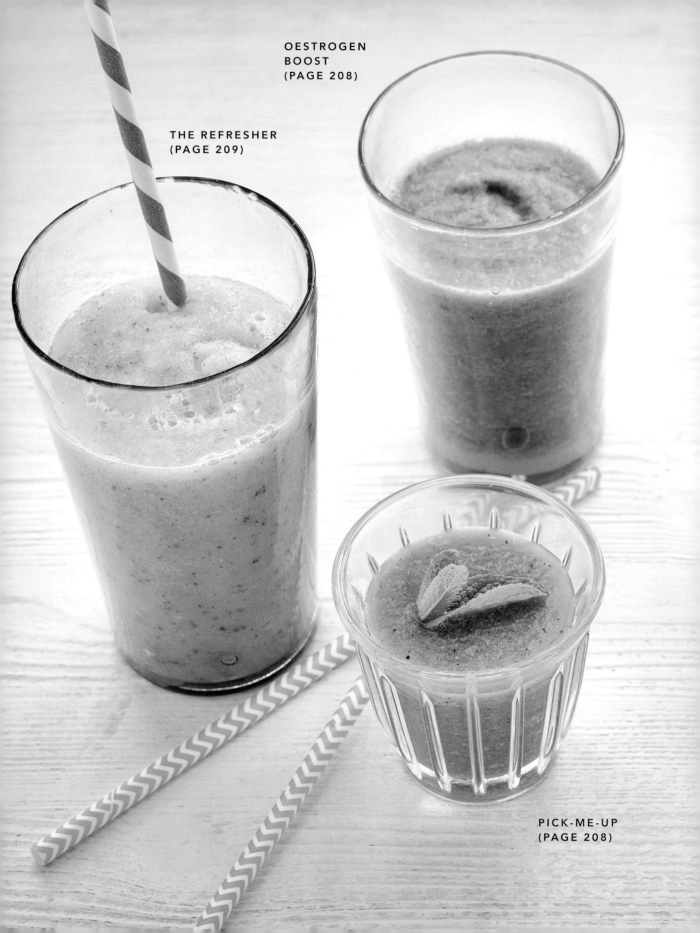

OESTROGEN
BOOST
(PAGE 208)

THE REFRESHER
(PAGE 209)

PICK-ME-UP
(PAGE 208)

GREEN OMEGA
(PAGE 209)

GLOWING NUTTY
(PAGE 209)

BREAKFAST
ON THE GO
(PAGE 209)

ALMOND MILK AND HAZELNUT HOT CHOCOLATE

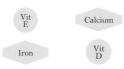

This velvety and comforting hot drink will make you feel instantly better from the inside out. It's like a hug in a mug on a cold night. It's also great as a smoothie if you whizz a banana up in it and serve it cold!

250ml almond milk, hazelnut milk or semi-skimmed cows' milk
1 heaped tbsp hazelnut-chocolate spread
1 tsp runny honey
pinch of ground cinnamon

1 Put all the ingredients in a small saucepan over a low heat. Whisk well until the hazelnut spread has melted into the hot milk. Bring to the boil, then simmer for 1 minute before serving in a large mug.

2 Enjoy with a Peanut Butter, Banana and Oatmeal Cookie (page 191).

VIRGIN HOT TODDY

This is the ideal drink to have if you are feeling like you may be coming down with a cold, have a cold or you feel as though your immune system could do with a little boost. My nan was the queen of making them for me when I was a little girl. This is her recipe adapted for pregnancy or for kids, and it's delicious. The ginger will help with any nausea as well as being healing for the throat. The honey will also help with this, as well as providing anti-inflammatory and anti-bacterial qualities. Lemon will provide you with a hit of vitamin C and is good for digestion. You can also add a decaffeinated Earl Grey tea bag along with the other ingredients for a stronger, more flavourful, drink if you wish.

1 tbsp runny honey
2cm piece fresh ginger, peeled and chopped into matchsticks
juice of ½ lemon
1 clove

Put all the ingredients in a small saucepan with 250ml cold water and bring to the boil over a high heat. Simmer for 1–2 minutes before straining into a large mug.

MULLED APPLE, CINNAMON AND ANISE

This is a great winter drink to enjoy when everyone else is drinking mulled wine and cider and you have to stick to the non-alcoholic tipples. It's delicious, warming and if you have to substitute mulled wine for anything, then this is it. This recipe serves 4–6, as it's better to make a batch. I'm sure you'll have a few takers: the designated drivers and of course the kiddies will welcome it.

SERVES 4–6

2 clementines, halved
3 cloves
1 litre pressed apple juice (pear juice also works well)
1 cinnamon stick
1 vanilla pod, split lengthways
1 star anise
2 eating apples (Royal Gala or Pink Lady are great), peeled and cut into 2cm chunks (you can also use pears)

Pierce the clementines with the cloves. Put all the ingredients in a saucepan and bring to the boil over a medium heat. Reduce the heat and simmer gently for 10 minutes. When the apples have started to soften, remove the clementine halves, and serve. I leave the spices in as they look so lovely. Reheat when you need a top-up.

FULL-TERM TEA

Raspberry leaf tea is said to soften the cervix and help with an easier delivery. Drink 2–3 cups per day.

ONLY DRINK WHEN AT TERM, FROM 37 WEEKS

3 tsp loose raspberry leaf tea
5cm piece fresh ginger, peeled
10 fresh mint leaves, plus extra to serve
2 tbsp fresh raspberries
juice of 1 lemon
1 tbsp agave nectar

Boil 200ml water and add 2 teaspoons of the loose tea leaves. Allow to infuse for 3 minutes before straining and keep the infused water. Now place the tea leaves, ginger, mint, raspberries, lemon juice and agave nectar into a blender and blitz until smooth. Add the infused tea and blend again. Strain once more, removing any bits. Pour over ice, add a little more fresh mint and enjoy. I suggest making a batch of this and keeping it chilled in the fridge once at term.

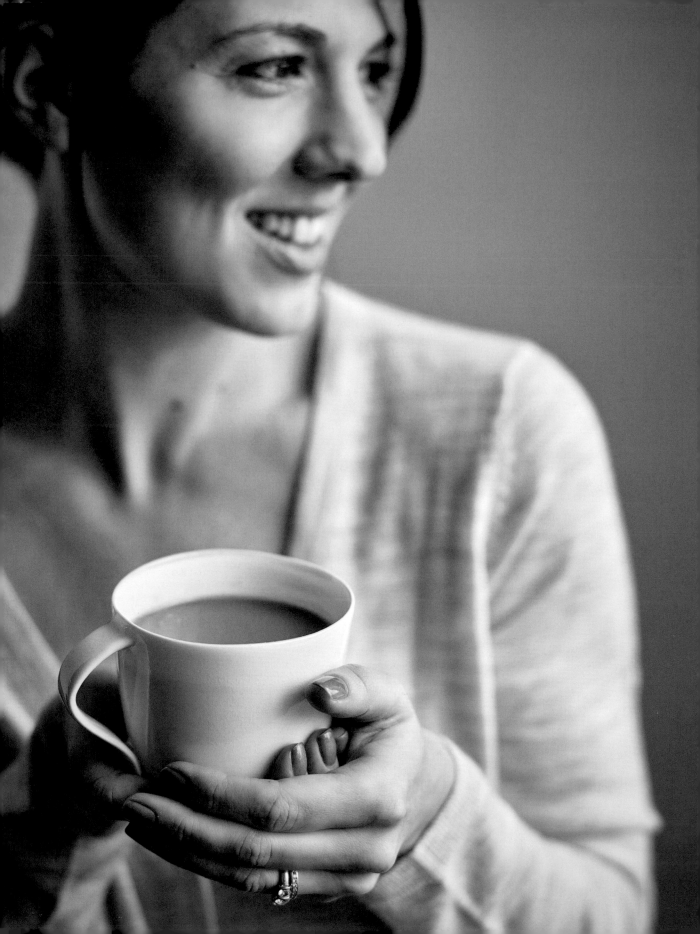

INDEX

Acknowledgements

To my amazing husband Tom: thank you! For always believing in me, supporting me and, of course, for rubbing my swollen feet during my pregnancy when no one else would. You are an incredible dad to Bertie. He simply adores you. Every day I tell myself how lucky we are to have you. We both love you so very much.

Mum, you have taught me how to be a mumma, helped and guided me through my pregnancy and now cherish and wholeheartedly love my Bertie. I can't tell you the joy it gives me to watch the two of you together and the special relationship you have built between nanny and grandson. Thank you for always being on call to recipe test, batch cook and even wash up when I simply didn't have the energy.

To my kind and generous mother-in-law Carol, for looking after B so lovingly at such a tiny age while I lost myself in the dreaded edits of *Blooming Delicious*, and for always having a spare bowl of soup and copious cups of decaf tea! We are so very lucky to have you and I am blessed to have married into such a wonderful family.

Thank you to my commissioning editor, Sam Jackson, for being so honest and for making *Blooming Delicious* come to life. It has been a pleasure to work with such a professional.

To my editor, Laura Herring, who just got it (every time!) and kept on pushing me to make *Blooming Delicious* even better.

To Henrietta, aka superwoman. I honestly don't know how you find enough hours in the day to be such a wonderful mum to three beautiful boys, run a very successful business, write books and still have time to spend on *Blooming Delicious*. Without you this book wouldn't have happened. Thank you for working with me and for all your help along the way.

To my wonderful photographer, Chris Terry, for making the recipes jump from the pages and for making the shoot days such a joyful breeze.

Thank you to the cool, calm and collected Rachel Wood, our food stylist, for being so enthusiastic about the book, cooking such delicious and beautiful food and for all the yummy lunches every day on the shoot.

And, finally, thank you to the design team at Smith & Gilmour who took *Blooming Delicious* from a rather flat looking text document and turned it into the book that you have just read. You have made it accessible, fun and easy to read.

You have all contributed in such special ways to helping me write this lovely book, which in turn I hope will help so many women eat well, be inspired and stay healthy on their exciting pregnancy journeys.

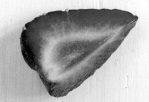

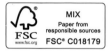
The information in this book has been compiled by way of general guidance in relation to the
specific subjects addressed, but is not a substitute and not to be relied on for medical, healthcare,
pharmaceutical or other professional advice on specific circumstances and in specific locations.
So far as the author is aware the information given is correct and up to date as at March 2016.
Practice, laws and regulations all change, and the reader should obtain up to date professional
advice on any such issues. The author and publishers disclaim, as far as the law allows, any liability
arising directly or indirectly from the use, or misuse, of the information contained in this book.

Footnotes

i. Lassi, Z.S. et al. (2014), 'Preconception care:
caffeine, smoking, alcohol, drugs and other
environmental chemical/radiation exposure',
Reproductive Health, Sept., 26 (11) Suppl: 3:S6.

ii. Greenwood, D.C. et al. (2014), 'Caffeine intake during
pregnancy and adverse birth outcomes: a systematic
review and dose-response meta-analysis', *European
Journal of Epidemiology*, Oct., 29(10):725–34.

iii. Mascarenhas, M. et al.(2014), 'Revisiting the role of
first trimester homocysteine as an index of maternal
and fetal outcome', *Journal of Pregnancy*,
2014:123024.

iv. Gagné, A. et al. (2009), 'Absorption, transport, and
bioavailability of vitamin E and its role in pregnant
women', *Journal of Obstetrics & Gynaecology
Canada*, 31(3):210–7.

v. Ruder, E.H. et al. (2014), 'Female dietary
antioxidant intake and time to pregnancy among
couples treated for unexplained infertility', *Fertility
& Sterility* 101(3):759–66.

vi. Hovdenak, N. et al. (2012), 'Influence of mineral
and vitamin supplements on pregnancy outcome',
*European Journal of Obstetrics, Gynecology &
Reproductive Biology*, 164(2):127–32.

vii. Palini, S. et al. (2014), 'Influence of ovarian
stimulation for IVF/ICSI on the antioxidant defence
system and relationship to outcome', *Reproductive
Biomedicine Online*, 29(1):65–71.

viii. Pieczyńska, J. et al. (2015), 'The role of selenium
in human conception and pregnancy', *Journal of
Trace Elements in Medicine and Biology*, 29C:31–38.